THE POCKET GUIDE FOR HIV AND AIDS NURSING CARE

Ansie Minnaar and Candice Bodkin

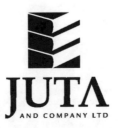

JUTA
AND COMPANY LTD

The Pocket Guide for HIV and AIDS Nursing Care
First published 2006 by
Juta & Co.
Mercury Crescent
Wetton, 7780
Cape Town, South Africa

© 2006 Juta & Co. Ltd

ISBN 10 digit: 0 7021 7193 X
ISBN 13 digit: 978 0721 71932

Typeset in 9/10 URWGrotesk

Project Manager: Sarah O'Neill
Editor: Dr Bridget Farham
Proofreader: Ethné Clarke
Indexer: Cecily van Gend
Typesetter: WaterBerry Designs cc
Cover designer: Alexander Kononov
Printed in South Africa by Creda Communications

CONTENTS

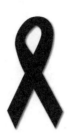

CONTRIBUTORS

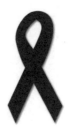

Ansie Minnaar PhD, RN, RM, RIN, RT, RNA is a senior lecturer at the University of the Witwatersrand, Johannesburg and holds a PhD (Natal), Community and Development. She also holds an MA Cur (Unisa) and BA Cur (Hons) (Unisa). She is also qualified in Intensive Care Nursing, with many years of experience in infection control and nosocomial infections and is currently involved in a research project: HIV and AIDS in nursing in the Gauteng area.

Candice Bodkin PhD, holds a BSc (Wits) in Genetics and Advanced Biology, an Advanced Diploma in Aromatherapy (School of Reflexology and Beauty), a B Nursing (Wits), an MSc (Wits) in Community Health, an Advanced Diploma in Nursing Education (Wits), a PhD (Wits) and a Diploma in Advanced Midwifery and Neonatal Nursing from RAU. She is currently a student, studying towards an MBBCh.

We dedicate this book to Angie and all nurses suffering as a result of the HIV & AIDS epidemic in South Africa.

PREFACE

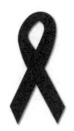

When the majority of mankind
is ravaged by HIV & AIDS...
all our lives
will be dramatically changed

(Richard Sowell 2005)

By the end of 2005, 65 million people worldwide were infected with HIV and AIDS. Half were under 25 years old, most of whom will die before the age of 35. One in four sexually active persons in South Africa is infected. AIDS is not a disease; it is a development disaster. The nursing curriculum needs to be changed so that HIV and AIDS are included in the main curriculum. The nursing profession in South Africa is in crisis, both because of the high number of patients dying of HIV and AIDS and because nurses themselves are infected with the virus. This book is written as a quick reference book for nurses across Africa who are nursing HIV and AIDS patients. It covers the medical and social aspects of the disease, as well as workplace issues, home-based care and palliative care.

SECTION 1

Chapter 1 is an introduction to the way that the virus is transmitted and how its transmission can be prevented. Voluntary counselling and testing are also covered, as is diagnosis.

Chapter 2 discusses the natural history of HIV infection, its signs and symptoms and how the infection is staged.

Chapter 3 discusses the opportunistic infections that are common in HIV and those that define AIDS, and how they are managed.

Chapter 4 introduces antiretroviral therapy in adults, including the three main drug classes, their mechanism of action, drug interactions, dosage schedules and side effects, concentrating on the treatment recommended in South Africa. Adherence counselling will also be addressed.

Chapter 5 covers an approach to the control of the nosocomial infections that are most important for HIV patients admitted to hospital. General infection control measures are covered.

Chapter 6 discusses the importance of lifestyle for the general health of those infected with HIV and outlines positive approaches to living with the virus that can improve overall health and slow down progression of the disease.

Chapter 7 covers complementary and alternative medicines (CAM). Many HIV patients use CAMs, so it is important to understand those that are most commonly used. Interactions between CAM and conventional medicines used in HIV are discussed, as are the potential risks and benefits of CAM in the management of HIV. Nutrition in HIV is discussed in detail.

SECTION 2

Chapter 8 discusses women and HIV and AIDS, the group most affected across southern Africa. This chapter discusses the reasons for increased infection rates in women and how these can be mitigated.

Chapter 9 discusses issues that are specific to the pregnant HIV positive woman, as well as the prevention of mother-to-child transmission of HIV (PMTCT) through the use of antiretroviral drugs, prevention measures during delivery and breastfeeding versus replacement feeding.

Chapter 10 covers the diagnosis of HIV in neonates and infants as well as the management of HIV infected children. This includes antiretroviral regimes and the treatment of opportunistic infections.

Chapter 11 looks at HIV and AIDS in the workplace. The increase in numbers of HIV positive patients in hospital means that nurses are more likely to come into contact with infected body fluids. The issues surrounding possible exposure to HIV and post-exposure prophylaxis are covered in detail.

SECTION 3

Chapter 12 discusses HIV and AIDS patients and critical care nursing. HIV is no longer a criteria used to determine whether or not to admit to intensive care units (ICU). This means that the illnesses seen in HIV patients in ICU and their management have changed over the years. Issues around ICU management of HIV positive patients are covered, as are the specific reasons for ICU admission, including adverse drug reactions.

Chapter 13 looks at home-based nursing care. Because of lack of access to antiretrovirals and difficulties in admitting all AIDS patients either to hospital or hospice, home-based care is becoming more important in the management of HIV and AIDS in southern Africa. This chapter covers what is provided by home based care and how carers should be trained.

Chapter 14 discusses palliative care. Many people infected with HIV will eventually require end-of-life care, either because they had no access to antiretrovirals, or because this treatment failed. The principles of palliative care are covered, as are specific issues such as pain and symptom control and spiritual and emotional care.

The appendix gives an overview of the epidemiology of HIV. Sub-Saharan Africa has the highest number of people living with HIV globally. In South Africa in 2004, there were 5.1 million people with the virus.

Ansie Minnaar and Candice Bodkin
Department of Nursing Education
University of the Witwatersrand
May 2006

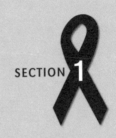

SECTION 1

TRANSMISSION, PREVENTION OF THE SPREAD OF HIV AND AIDS AND VOLUNTARY COUNSELLING AND TESTING (VCT)

Ansie Minnaar

KEY CONCEPTS

- basic awareness
- immune system
- transmission
- counselling
- VCT, CTR
- complications and opportunistic infection

- drug regimens
- effective communication
- primary, secondary and tertiary prevention of HIV infection
- behavioural change
- ethical and legal, prevention of transmission of HIV

PREAMBLE

Imagine your life this way...

You wake up in the morning and have your breakfast with your two kids. They are already doomed to die in infancy. Your husband, who works away from home, comes home twice a month and sleeps around in between. You know that you are risking your life in every act of sexual intercourse with him. On your way to work you pass a house where a teenager lives alone taking care of the other young

children, without any source of income. At another house,
the wife was called a prostitute, beaten and thrown into
the streets when she asked her husband to use a condom.
Over there, on the pavement, lies a man desperately sick,
without access to a doctor, clinic, medicine, food, blankets
or even a kind word. At work you drink tea with colleagues,
and every third one is already fatally ill and is not really
coping with the workload anymore... You whisper about a
friend who went for VCT and disclosed her HIV status...
and whose neighbours stoned her to death. Your leisure
and time off is occupied by the funerals you attend every
Saturday. You and your neighbours and your political and
popular leaders act as though nothing is happening...

Can you and your organisation afford to ignore this threat?

PRE-TEST: HOW MUCH DO YOU KNOW ABOUT HIV AND AIDS?

HIV and AIDS Survey

1 What does the word AIDS stand for?

A	_____	3
I	_____	3
D	_____	3
S	_____	3

	Item	Yes	No	Maybe
2	Does HIV cause AIDS?			
3	Where did AIDS originate?			
a	Africa			
b	America			
c	Monkeys			
d	Sex with homosexuals			

	Item	Yes	No	Maybe
e	Sex with witches			
4	Is HIV inflicted on humankind as a punishment for the wicked?			
5	Can you tell that someone has HIV infection just by looking at them?			
6	Can someone who is HIV-positive pass the virus on to his/her partner?			
7	Can you get infected with HIV from kissing?			
8	Can you get infected with HIV from shaking hands with an HIV-positive person?			
9	Can you get infected with HIV by using the same toilet as an infected person?			
10	Can you get infected with HIV by someone who is not HIV-positive?			
11	Can you get infected with HIV by a mosquito?			
12	Can you get infected with HIV from intercourse with an HIV-infected person?			
13	Are all children of HIV-infected mothers at risk of becoming HIV-positive?			
14	Can a child get HIV from their HIV-positive mother's breast milk?			
15	Can you get AIDS from caring for AIDS patients?			
16	Is the HIV test performed at the doctor's surgery?			
17	Does using a condom properly lower the risk of HIV infection?			
18	Does using a condom properly lower the risk of being infected with a sexually transmitted infection?			
19	Can we treat HIV infection?			

	Item	Yes	No	Maybe
20	Can doctors treat HIV infection?			
21	Are AIDS and HIV infection gay diseases?			
22	Can you cure HIV infections by having unprotected sex with a virgin girl or boy?			
23	Do you think HIV and AIDS will solve the unemployment problem in South Africa?			
24	Do you think HIV and AIDS is someone else's problem and not your own?			
25	Do you think that someone with HIV/AIDS can also have tuberculosis (TB)?			
26	Do you think that someone with TB always has HIV and AIDS?			
27	Do you think HIV-positive people should have sex?			
28	If you were HIV-positive or have AIDS, would you tell your sexual partner?			
29	Do you know your HIV status?			

Each correct answer counts 3 marks

Calculate your mark: / 114x 100   %

(Answers on page 22)

In a few words, can you tell us what you think we should do about preventing HIV and AIDS?

_____

_____

_____

_____

_____

_____

_____

INTRODUCTION

Sexual contact is the main way that HIV is transmitted in most parts of the world. HIV can be transmitted by a man or a woman. The highest risk behaviour is receptive intercourse, either anal or vaginal, without a condom. The greater the number of sexual partners a person has, the greater their risk of exposure to HIV.

TRANSMISSION OF HIV

HIV is transmitted through body fluids and through blood products. The main modes of transmission are:

* unprotected sexual intercourse, vaginal or anal
* through contaminated blood or blood products
* from mother to child, either through the placenta before delivery, during delivery or through breast milk
* during sharing of needles by drug users
* rarely, as a result of percutaneous needle stick injury or mucosal blood splash.

The risk of infection from blood products in South Africa is small as all blood donations are routinely screened for HIV using sensitive and specific assays, and donors who are regarded as high risk are excluded from donating when they fill out questionnaires asking about their risk of acquiring HIV.

Sharing of contaminated needles, including those used for injecting steroids and insulin, but mainly for illegal injected drugs, is also a common mode of HIV transmission and is the second highest cause of HIV infection in the United States. The sexual partners and unborn children of infected injection drug users contract HIV through secondary transmission.

Strategies to prevent spread of infection from injection drug users include the following:

* treatment for substance abuse and provision of sterile needles and syringes for those who continue to use drugs
* needle exchange programmes and instructions on how to clean needles using a 10% solution of household bleach
* distribution of condoms.

It is unlikely that an effective vaccine against HIV infection will be widely available in the next ten years. Other therapies such as antiretroviral therapy are still not widely available, so behavioural change remains the most viable way of limiting the spread of HIV infection. There are three major classes of programmes to prevent sexual transmission (*Harrison et al. 2000*) of HIV:

1. HIV counselling and testing – called voluntary counselling and testing (VCT)
2. Individual and community sexual risk reduction interventions to promote safer sex
3. Biomedical approaches to prevent sexual transmission, such as the use of antiretroviral drugs to prevent infections in persons exposed to HIV (post-exposure prophylaxis) (*Farnham et al. 2002*).

HIV VOLUNTARY COUNSELLING AND TESTING (VCT)

Knowing your HIV status is the most important way to stop the spread of the virus. Voluntary counselling and testing (VCT) programmes are an essential part of this. This is particularly the case now that antiretroviral treatment that can prevent progression of the infection and be used as post-exposure prophylaxis is available. An HIV test may also be in the interests of a third person; for example after a needle stick injury or for a pregnant woman wishing to protect her unborn child. An HIV test should never be performed without the informed consent of the patient, pre-test counselling and an arrangement made for post-test follow-up and counselling.

HIV antibody diagnosis

Antibody tests are the most commonly used HIV tests. Two different enzyme-linked immunosorbent assay (ELISA) tests or two different rapid tests (on site) to confirm HIV infection meet the World Health Organisation (WHO) testing recommendations for countries such as South Africa, where HIV prevalence is more than 10%.

ELISA screening test

The ELISA test is the most widely used serological technique today. These tests have been used since the early 1990s. The ELISA for the HIV antibody uses the HIV antigen to capture HIV antibodies in a blood sample, which is fixed to a plastic well in a multi-well plate. The second step detects captured antibody using an enzyme-substrate colour reaction. Today, large laboratories run fully automatic ELIZA systems.

False positive HIV antibody tests

False positive tests can arise as a result of the inherent characteristics of the test system. Examples of cross-reacting antibodies are numerous and are found in various clinical settings including autoimmune diseases, in pregnancy, in a variety of acute infections and in people taking part in clinical trials of HIV vaccines. A distinguishing feature of these cross-reactions is that they usually cause low-level or borderline positivity. Confirmatory testing will usually confirm whether or not the test is positive.

Rapid tests

Rapid HIV tests are easy to use and make it possible to provide test results at the time that the test is done. Rapid tests are usually indicated for patients who are unlikely to return for test results, in emergency departments, and for pregnant women in labour who have not previously been tested. Two tests are needed for confirmation of HIV infection.

Urine tests

Calypte Biomedical Corp.'s HIV-1 Urine EIA is the only FDA-approved urine test. Only a healthcare provider can perform this test, and positive results must be confirmed. Testing with urine limits blood-borne pathogen exposure for healthcare workers. There are no urine tests available in South Africa.

HI virus testing

Specific tests for HIV antigen, DNA, RNA or viral culture are additional methods used to detect HIV infection. Viral cultures are very expensive and labour intensive and are mainly used for viral isolation for analysis or for HIV detection in infants. DNA PCR (polymerase chain reaction) tests are used in South Africa for the diagnosis of HIV in infants. They can also be used in the window period when normal antibody testing does not detect HIV infection.

Monitoring immune function

The viral load and the CD4 cell count are the standard tests used to evaluate the status of the immune system and are also used to predict the prognosis of HIV infection. The viral load predicts the rate of disease progression (rate of loss of CD4 cells) and the CD4 count indicates the stage of disease that the patient has already reached. The CD4 cell percentage is used in preference to the CD4 count in children because normal CD4 counts are age-dependent. In adults normal values for CD4 cell counts range from 800 to 1050 cells/μl with a standard deviation of 500 to 1300 cells/μl. CD4 cell counts may also be a surrogate marker for HIV infection in patients who refuse to be tested, as there are few other conditions associated with severe depletion of CD4 cell counts. Therefore, a patient with either a low CD4 cell count or one of the AIDS-defining diseases is likely to have HIV infection and should be strongly counselled regarding HIV testing. CD4 testing should be carried out regularly, particularly once a patient is on treatment. In South Africa, CD4 testing is recommended before starting antiretroviral therapy and every four to six months thereafter.

Significant exposure

Significant exposure to HIV occurs when medical or non-medical personnel are exposed to blood or other potentially infectious materials during the performance of their job. This occurs as a result of a needle stick injury (sharps and needles), a splash to mucous membranes, contact with non-intact skin or contact with intact skin that is extensive or prolonged. Medical personnel have the right to know the HIV status of the source patient involved in the exposure, but the source patient must be asked to consent to the test. The legal situation in South Africa if the source patient refuses consent is not clear. But there have been cases where blood from previous samples has been tested without the source patient's consent.

Advantages and disadvantages of HIV testing

Advantages	Disadvantages
Earlier medical treatment so prolonging life	May get a false negative result
Reduced anxiety and acceptance of infection	Increased anxiety about the effects of the infection
Decreased chance of transmission to others if behaviour changes	May abuse drugs or attempt suicide
Decreased chance of re-infection with a different strain of the virus if behaviour changes	Subjected to stigma by community
Lifestyle and behaviour changes	Confidentiality issues
Increased knowledge of HIV	Difficulty in obtaining life insurance
	Problems with dealing with a relationship or partner

Table 1.1

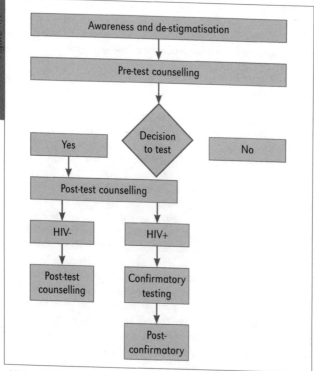

HIV and AIDS testing

COUNSELLING

One of the goals of counselling is to determine the patient's level of risk of exposure and to encourage voluntary testing if the patient is at high risk. Risks for HIV exposure include: multiple sexual partners, substance abuse, needle sharing, partners with HIV, a history of sexually transmitted infections (STI), children of an HIV-positive mother, a history of sexual assault or domestic violence, sex for drugs or money, a history of transfusion of blood/blood products or transplants and occupational exposure. Risk should not be evaluated on the basis of age, religion, sexual orientation, gender, race/ethnicity, marital status or social/economic/cultural factors.

Pre-test counselling must take into consideration the patient's intellectual capacity, age, language skills and their culture when explaining the testing process. Counselling must include the reason for the test and how it will be done, information on how HIV is transmitted and how exposure to HIV can be prevented and options for eliminating or reducing high-risk behaviours.

INFORMED CONSENT

An HIV test must be voluntary and cannot be performed without the informed consent of the patient or his/her legal representative. Consent for general treatment does not meet the requirement for informed consent for HIV testing. The patient may withdraw informed consent at any time. A patient cannot give informed consent if they are under the influence of drugs and/or alcohol or do not understand the information. To encourage testing in adolescents, minors, under the age of 18, may give informed consent for HIV testing (or any STI) without their parent's knowledge. The healthcare provider has the discretion to determine if a minor has the intellectual capacity to understand HIV testing. Parents are not to be notified of test results either directly or indirectly unless this is authorised in writing by the minor. When obtaining informed consent, the test procedure, the limitations of the test and confidentiality must be explained to the patient. Make arrangements for follow-up to report the results of the test and for post-test counselling. Make it clear to the patient that the result is absolutely confidential and will not be reported to anyone else without his or her consent (*HIV/AIDS Update 2004*).

HIV COUNSELLING – A PRACTICAL APPROACH

Ideally, every patient who wants HIV testing should be fully counselled by a professionally trained counsellor. However, in South Africa, this is often not practical or possible, so nurses need to understand HIV counselling. In most cases, the counselling will be carried out by the nurse or doctor who has asked for a patient's HIV test. Wherever possible, the same person should then give the patient the result and be available for post-test counselling.

The aims of HIV counselling are to:

- Provide support.
- Help patients with issues and problems around HIV testing.
- Explore a patient's current coping skills and help them to develop new ones.

- Help patients to become self-sufficient.
- Provide information to HIV-negative patients that will allow them to remain HIV-negative.
- Provide information to HIV-positive patients that will allow them to avoid re-infection and to prevent them from infecting others.
- Discuss behaviour change.
- Give information on HIV services and other related services available to the patient.

HIV prevention counselling should focus on the patient's own needs and unique circumstances and risks. The counselling should be face to face and should last around 15 to 20 minutes. Emphasise prevention by focusing on HIV risk reduction in a way that is relevent to each patient. This includes an in-depth, personalised risk assessment to explore previous risk-reduction efforts and to identify any successful risk behaviour interventions. Use the session to acknowledge and provide support for positive steps towards reduction of high-risk behaviour on the side of the patient as this is an important step in reducing risks.

Clarify critical misconceptions regarding the transmission of HIV and emphasise substantial risks rather than minimal risks, although these should also be discussed. Negotiate a concrete, achievable behaviour-change step that will reduce the risk of HIV infection or transmission. Small behavioural changes can reduce the probability of acquiring or transmitting the virus. For many patients, knowledge of their partners' recent HIV status is more important to them than personal behaviour changes. Be flexible and use the opportunity to provide information about using condoms, male and female, and the risks of needle sharing, although this is not yet common in South Africa. Use explicit and simple language when giving test results.

Counsellors need special skills, training and updates on HIV and AIDS. Effective HIV counselling includes:

- completion of the standard training course in patient/client centred HIV prevention counselling
- belief that counselling can make a difference
- genuine interest in the counselling process
- the ability to use active listening skills and a willingness to listen to patients
- the ability to use open-ended questions
- the ability to comfort patients with an interactive and persuasive approach

- supplying a supportive and trusting atmosphere in the counselling process
- being interested in learning new counselling and skill-building techniques
- being informed and up to date with new developments regarding the risk of HIV transmission
- being comfortable in discussions on specific HIV risk behaviours, such as unsafe sex or needle sharing
- being able to remain focused on risk reduction strategies
- supporting quality improvement measures.

Principles of HIV counselling, testing and referral (CTR)

- **Protect the confidentiality of patients who are recommended to or receive HIV CTR services.** Personal information should not be discussed without the patient's consent.
- **Obtain informed consent before HIV testing.** HIV testing should be voluntary and free of choice. Information regarding consent may be presented orally or in writing and should be recorded. Accepting or refusing testing should not have detrimental consequences on the quality of care offered to patients.
- **Provide patients with the option of anonymous HIV testing.** Anonymous testing can benefit the health of individuals and the community. People who would not otherwise be tested might seek anonymous HIV testing and learn about safer sexual practices and how to prevent the spread of HIV.
- **Provide information on the HIV test to all who are sent for testing, whether or not prevention counselling is provided.** The information should include what HIV test results mean.
- **Adhere to legal requirements and government policies governing HIV.** Information on services, policies, funding and the provision of grants must be given to patients.
- **Provide services that are responsive to client and community needs and priorities.** Provide information on services and ways of accessing these services, for example community-based or outreach services.
- **Provide services that are appropriate to the client's culture, language, sex and sexual orientation.** Provide services that increase the likelihood that a patient will return for test results.
- Ensure high-quality services. Ensure ongoing, high-quality services that serve the patient in a humane manner. Furthermore, implement written protocols for CTR and written reports of quality improvement and evaluation processes (*Divine et al. 2001*).

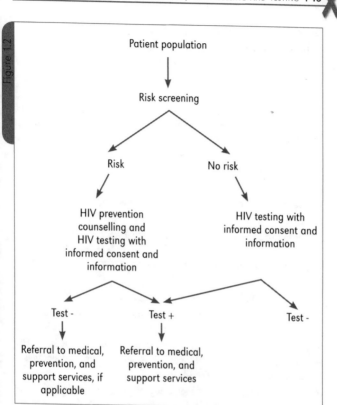

Example of CTR in high -prevalence settings

Source: Divine, Greby, Hunt, Kamb, Steketee & Warner 2001

How to evaluate the patient's risk of HIV infection

The nurse could ask an open-ended question such as: 'What are you doing now or what have you done in the past that you think may put you at risk for HIV infection?'

A checklist or a self-administered questionnaire, computer-assisted interview or any other instrument can be used for screening. An example is provided on the next page.

Example of a risk screening questionnaire.

Instruction: Please tick applicable phrases:

The opening remark could be, for example: *Since your last HIV test (if ever), have you:*

1. Injected drugs and shared equipment (e.g. needles, syringes) with others?
2. Had unprotected intercourse with someone that you think might be infected (e.g. a partner who injected drugs, has been diagnosed or treated for an STI or hepatitis, has had multiple or anonymous sex partners, or who has exchanged sex for drugs or money)?
3. Had unprotected vaginal or anal intercourse with more than one sex partner?
4. Been diagnosed or treated for an STI, hepatitis, or TB?
5. Had a fever or illness of unknown cause?
6. Been told you have an infection related to a weak immune system?

Patients who should be recommended to attend HIV prevention CTR

The following patients should be recommended to attend CTR:

- All patients in settings that serve populations at increased behavioural or clinical risk of HIV.
- All patients who have clinical signs or symptoms suggesting HIV infection such as fever or illness of unknown origin or opportunistic infections, including active TB.
- All patients who have diagnoses suggesting an increased risk of HIV infection such as another STI.
- All patients who self-report HIV risks.
- All patients who attend clinics in areas of high HIV prevalence.
- Regardless of HIV prevalence in the area or behavioural or clinical risk the following patients should be recommended to attend CTR:
  - all pregnant women
  - all patients with possible acute occupational exposure
  - all patients with known sexual or needle-sharing exposure.

Useful questions which could aid in patient-centred HIV prevention counselling

Open-ended questions could assist the HIV counsellor in establishing the patient's behavioural risks, for example:

- What are you doing that you think may be putting you at risk for HIV infection?
- What are the riskiest things that you are doing?
- If your test comes back positive, how do you think you may have become infected?
- When was the last time you put yourself at risk for HIV? What happened?
- How often do you use drugs or alcohol?
- How do you think that drugs or alcohol may influence your risk of HIV infection?
- How often do you use condoms when you have sex?
- When and with whom do you have sex without a condom? When and with whom do you have sex with a condom?
- What are you currently doing to protect yourself from HIV? How is that working?
- What kinds of things do you do to protect your partner from being infected with HIV?
- Tell me about specific situations when you have reduced your HIV risk. How was that possible?
- How risky are your sex/drug use patterns?
- Have you recently been tested for HIV? (*Divine et al. 2001*).

Populations at increased behavioural or clinical risk for HIV infection

HIV prevention and CTR should be routinely recommended for all patients in settings where the patient population is at increased risk of acquiring or transmitting HIV. In these settings patients with ongoing risk behaviour should be linked to additional HIV prevention treatment such as counselling, condoms and, where applicable, access to clean needles and syringes. Places where populations may be at increased behavioural or clinical risk of HIV infection include:

- adolescent or school-based health clinics with high rates of STIs
- clinics serving men who have sex with men
- correctional services, prisons, juvenile detention centres
- drug or alcohol prevention and treatment programmes
- freestanding HIV test sites
- homeless shelters

- outreach programmes
- STI clinics
- TB clinics.

POST-TEST COUNSELLING GUIDELINES

Knowledge of HIV status is a critical HIV prevention strategy and essential for entry into antiretroviral programmes. A plan must be developed that encourages patients to return to receive their results. Wherever possible, results should not be given over the phone, particularly a positive result. However, patients can be contacted by phone to make follow-up and counselling appointments. Rapid testing generally ensures that patients receive their test results, as the result is provided on the same day as the test.

The following information is important when considering HIV testing:

- There is a delay between becoming infected with HIV and HIV antibodies being detectable in the blood. This is called the window period. A patient may need to return for a repeat test if there is a possibility that he or she is in the window period of infection. Prevention counselling is important during this period.
- Most infected persons will develop detectable HIV antibodies within three months of exposure. Therefore a second repeat test should be considered within six to12 months after exposure if the first test is negative.
- Ongoing exposure causes a continued risk of HIV infection and is a special challenge for follow-up testing. Follow-up testing monitors the patient's HIV status, and can also provide a platform for HIV prevention counselling and support.
- If there is no identifiable risk for HIV infection but patients come repeatedly for follow-up testing, this should regarded as an opportunity to provide in-depth prevention counselling and referral to support services.

SEXUAL RISK REDUCTION INTERVENTIONS AND COMMUNITY NORMS REGARDING SAFER SEX

Currently about one in four women attending antenatal clinics in South Africa is infected with HIV. South Africa is experiencing an explosive epidemic of HIV and AIDS. The highest incidence of HIV infection is in women between 15 and 30 years of age. There is good evidence that behaviour change interventions are effective in reducing high-risk behaviour. Communication, educating people about the nature of the epidemic and ways to prevent infection, condom promotion and behaviour change initiatives that encourage people to reduce the number of sexual partners can reduce high-risk sexual behaviour. Programmes that encourage delaying the age of first sex and abstinance from sex have also showed some success in young people.

However, in South Africa, in spite of these interventions, the HIV infection rate is still increasing. This suggests that these efforts have been too limited and are not effective. Future efforts should target high-risk groups, especially among women. Prevention programmes should aim at activities that empower young women to negotiate condom use and to make other decisions regarding their sexual relationships. Male or female condoms are the most effective way to prevent HIV infection during sex. Young men and women also need education and training on the gender imbalances among South African communities, because these are important in the way that HIV has spread in the community.

Most behaviour change interventions are based on cognitive-behavioural theories, emphasising the importance of group norms and collective change, as shown in the models below.

Theory of reasoned action

- Need for awareness of risk
- Acceptance of the risk
    - Acquisition of specific skills to reduce risk
    - Continuum that leads from attitude change, interventions to reduce risk, actual behaviour change.

Health belief model

Beliefs concerning susceptibility to risk eventually exceed a threshold and trigger action for change.

Bandura's social learning theory

Self-efficacy: An individual's belief in his/her own ability to perform risk-reducing behaviours in vulnerable situations. Action such as using condoms is determined by an understanding of what must be done to achieve such behaviour.

The AIDS-risk reduction model

- Individual self-description of being at risk
- Commitment to change through increasingly protective actions such as:
  - recognition of risk
  - commitment to change
  - acquisition of skills that can lead to help-seeking, condom use and other risk-reducing behaviour.

Specific risk-reduction steps

Specific risk-reduction steps in HIV prevention, which are more likely to be effective in changing behaviour, are as follows:

- Buy a condom today and try it on. (If female, try the female condom).
- Carry a condom next time you go out (clubbing).
- Starting today, put condoms at your bedside.
- Starting tonight, insist that either your partner uses a condom, or you won't participate in vaginal (or anal) sex.
- Stop seeing a partner who is seeing other people as well.
- Break up with a partner before going out with someone new.
- Talk honestly with your partner about HIV and ask about his/her HIV status.
- Avoid getting high on drugs and alcohol.
- Until you have both had an HIV test, only kiss.
- Ask your partner today if he/she has had a recent HIV test and has been tested for other STIs.
- Obtain clean needles and syringes before you use drugs again.
- Contact a drug rehabilitation centre.

(*Divine et al. 2001*).

CONTROLLING SEXUALLY TRANSMITTED INFECTIONS

The presence of STIs magnifies the risk of HIV transmission during unprotected sex as much as ten-fold. Most of these infections can be cured relatively easily with common antibiotic treatment. South Africa faces particular difficulties because of lack of services, poor availability of drugs, limited access to clinics and poverty. STIs are treated using syndromic management in South Africa. This involves recognising clinical signs and symptoms and prescribing treatment for the major STIs that cause these signs and symptoms. This allows health workers who lack specialised skills and access to laboratory tests to effectively treat most symptomatic infections during a patient's first clinic visit.

HSV-2 (Herpes simplex Virus-2) has been identified as a co-factor of HIV susceptibility in South Africa. HSV-2s co-occurrence with HIV indicates that HSV-2 control may be a valuable part of HIV prevention. The obstacle, however is that there is no cure for HSV-2 and vaccines are still not available. The infection is lifelong and ulcers will reappear periodically throughout an infected person's life. Treatment for the ulcers is expensive and testing for HSV-2 is difficult in poorer countries. Early sexual education and consistent condom use remain the best prevention.

THE WAY FORWARD

It is clear that young women, between the ages of 15 and 25 years, are at particularly high risk of infection. Determinants of risk for young women are gender inequality, a lack of power in decision making and sexual coercion. Behaviour intervention with specific goals for young women is needed. Other high-risk groups are male migrant workers and sex workers. Prevention programmes need to be targeted at these specific groups as well as the broader community.

Whilst condom use is heavily emphasised in South African prevention programmes, the correct use of condoms needs to be focussed upon.

It may be that condom use has been over-emphasised at the expense of other prevention messages, such as:

- reducing the number of unsafe partners
- having one faithful and safe partner
- abstaining from sex
- delaying the onset of sexual activities.

Dual protection against pregnancy and infection is an important message in risk reduction. Better distribution of resources may be a crucial determinant of HIV infection. Condoms are key to preventing the spread of HIV and AIDS and STIs. Condom programmes work best as part of a comprehensive package of intervention that includes HIV and AIDS education, sexual health and human sexuality, and gender sensitivity training.

STRATEGIC GOALS FOR THE COMPREHENSIVE PREVENTION OF HIV

Key elements in the comprehensive prevention of HIV are as follows:

- Introduction policies that help to reduce the vulnerability of large numbers of people, which include the creation of a social, legal and economic environment in which prevention is possible. This includes access to education, empowerment of women and cooperation in preventing human trafficking for sexual exploitation.
- Closing the prevention gap – less than one in five people have access to prevention services.
- Involving a wide range of interventions to combat the spread of HIV.
- Eliminating AIDS-related stigma and discrimination.
- Tailoring prevention strategies to meet the specific needs of people. Give special attention to vulnerable groups of people.

CONCLUSION

The key to preventing the transmission of HIV lies mainly in changing behaviour, since a vaccine against the virus is still a long way off. Anti-retroviral therapy (see Chapter 4) is effective in preventing the progression of the disease but is expensive and, as yet, still only available to a small number of people in South Africa.

ANSWERS TO PRE-TEST

1. A acquired	4. No	14. Yes	24. No
I immuno	5. No	15. No	25. Yes
D deficiency	6. Yes	16. Yes	26. No
S syndrome	7. No	17. Yes	27. No unprotected sex
2. Yes	8. No	18. No	
3a. Maybe	9. No	19. Yes	28. Yes
3b. No	10. No	20. Yes	29. Yes
3c. Yes	11. No	21. No	
3d. No	12. Yes	22. No	
3e. No	13. Yes	23. No	

CHAPTER 2

PATHOPHYSIOLOGY OF HIV AND AIDS

Candice Bodkin

> HIV/AIDS is the mirror in the face of our society. It forces us to examine the contours of our face as it really is, not as we would like to see it. Like any face ours bears the scars of the past, the impact of the realities of today and indications of how the future is likely to shape up for us
>
> (Mamphela Ramphele 2005)

INTRODUCTION

The human immunodeficiency virus (HIV) is a virus that infects immune cells causing a progressive decline in immune function. The immune system ultimately becomes so weak that the body succumbs to pathogens that would not normally cause illness and the HIV-positive person develops recurrent infections. Once the immune system is depleted to the extent that the person cannot evade infections, the individual is said to have acquired immunodeficiency syndrome (AIDS). These infections are called opportunistic infections and are AIDS-defining illnesses.

HIV belongs to the *Lentivirus* group of the retrovirus family. To date, two types of HIV virus have been identified. These are HIV-1 and HIV-2. HIV-1 is the most common cause of AIDS and is responsible for the global pandemic. HIV-2 infection is largely confined to West Africa with limited spread to other countries, and will also cause AIDS, but is generally a less severe infection.

Retroviruses characteristically contain the enzyme reverse transcriptase, which is responsible for the reverse transcription of single-stranded viral RNA into double-stranded DNA. Once the HI virus has produced viral DNA, it is able to incorporate its genetic material into the human DNA. The enzyme reverse transcriptase is the target site for the drugs called nucleoside reverse transcriptase inhibitors and non-nucleoside reverse transcriptase inhibitors.

HIV evolves rapidly because the process of reverse transcription is highly error prone and there is a high daily turnover of virus. This allows the virus to adapt rapidly and diversify, with serious implications for both drug treatment and the progression of the disease. Drug resistance develops rapidly and the virus can escape detection by the immune system, allowing spread through the body. Rapid development of drug resistance is the reason that HIV is treated with three or more drugs, because treatment with only one drug would allow rapid development of resistance (*Kumar & Clark 2004*).

HIV TRANSMISSION

As discussed in Chapter 1, HIV is transmitted:

- during unprotected sexual intercourse
- from mother to child during pregnancy, labour and breastfeeding
- during the sharing of needles by intravenous drug users
- rarely, from HIV-infected blood transfusion
- rarely, as a result of percutaneous needle stick injury or mucosal blood splash.

HIV is more likely to be transmitted in the following instances:

- In the presence of a high viral load and a low CD4 count. A high HIV viral load occurs during seroconversion illness, in patients with advanced HIV infection and in patients who are not adherent to antiretroviral therapy.

- HIV is more likely to be transmitted during rape or rough unprotected intercourse, as a result of genital trauma.

- HIV is more likely to be transmitted in the presence of a sexually transmitted infection, because genital ulceration or inflammation provides a point of access for the virus.

- HIV is more likely to be transmitted from mother to child in the presence of maternal infection, low maternal CD4 count and high viral load. Low birthweight babies and pre-term babies are more likely to contract HIV infection during pregnancy and labour.

- HIV is more likely to be transmitted from mother to child during breastfeeding if the mother has cracked nipples or the baby has oral thrush. Mixed breast and other feeding is also more likely to promote transmission of the virus because the child's gut may be damaged by other feeds, making it easier for the virus to penetrate.

THE NATURAL HISTORY OF HIV INFECTION

HIV and AIDS is caused by a virus that attaches to and destroys CD4 T-lymphocytes, which are integral to immune system functioning. This results in a gradual decline in immune function and increased susceptibility to invasion by opportunistic pathogens. Over time, the immune system is depleted, indicated by a decreasing CD4 count, and viral replication increases, indicated by an increasing viral load.

HIV infection

The HI virus initially infects specialised dendritic cells, also called Langerhans cells, which are present in the genital mucosa. Dendritic cells express high levels of CD4 and CCR5 which facilitate HIV infection. HIV virions are trapped in the dendritic cells and transported to the lymphoid tissue. Once in the lymphoid tissue the HIV virions begin to replicate and new virions are released from lymphoid tissue and spread to other parts of the body, including the central nervous system, via the blood. This is the start of primary HIV infection or seroconversion disease.

The HIV lifecycle

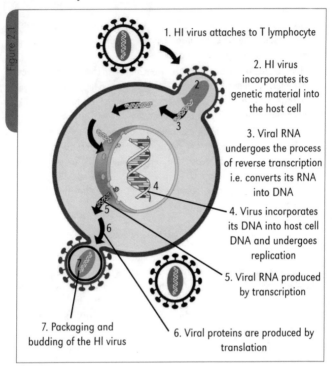

1. HI virus attaches to T lymphocyte

2. HI virus incorporates its genetic material into the host cell

3. Viral RNA undergoes the process of reverse transcription i.e. converts its RNA into DNA

4. Virus incorporates its DNA into host cell DNA and undergoes replication

5. Viral RNA produced by transcription

6. Viral proteins are produced by translation

7. Packaging and budding of the HI virus

The lifecycle of HIV

THE PROGRESSION OF HIV TO AIDS

HIV progresses through various stages that result in full-blown AIDS. About half of people newly infected with HIV will have a non-specific viral illness that is similar to infectious mononucleosis. This develops between one and six weeks after infection. This is called seroconversion illness.

An asymptomatic stage follows seroconversion illness. In those patients who did not experience a seroconversion illness, the infection is asymptomatic from the beginning. This asymptomatic stage may continue for up to ten years without treatment, depending on the immune status of the individual, until immune system breakdown occurs and the illnesses that are characteristic of AIDS start to develop.

Primary HIV infection/seroconversion disease

The initial event in HIV infection is acute HIV syndrome, also known as HIV seroconversion disease, which occurs in about 50% of those infected. This early stage is characterised by a decline in CD4 cell count and a high viral load, indicated by high concentrations of viral RNA in the plasma. Viral RNA shows an initial rise; this occurs at seroconversion. During acute HIV infection the viral load can be very high (10 million copies/ml of plasma) (*Wilson et al. 2002*). This high viral load makes the newly infected individual highly infectious. The high viral load stimulates the immune system to produce antibodies against viral proteins. Once this immune response develops, the viral load decreases and remains at a relatively stable set point viral load. This viral load set point is a point at which the production and clearance of viral particles by the immune system are equal and is specific for each individual. Clinical recovery from the seroconversion syndrome is accompanied by a reduction in viral RNA. Once the immune system has been stimulated to produce antibodies, the HIV test (such as the rapid HIV test or ELISA) becomes positive.

Acute HIV infection (seroconversion syndrome) is characterised by the following common symptoms:

- fever
- lymphadenopathy
- pharyngitis
- morbilliform rash
- mucocutaneous ulceration
- myalgia
- arthralgia.

Less common symptoms include:

- diarrhoea
- headache
- nausea
- vomiting
- hepatosplenomegaly
- oral candidiasis.

There is often widespread lymphadenopathy.

Seroconversion disease can occasionally be severe and last more than two weeks. An individual with severe seroconversion disease tends to have a higher set point viral load at the resolution of the acute HIV infection and this is associated with a poor prognosis.

The window period

After HIV transmission occurs there is a delay before HIV antibodies become detectable in the blood. This lasts about four weeks. However, tests for the virus itself will show the infection earlier. The P24 antigen test is positive in most patients before the ELISA test, which detects antibodies to HIV in the blood, will become positive. Polymerase chain reaction (PCR) testing will show HIV in the blood about two weeks after infection.

Asymptomatic infection

During this stage the HIV-positive person shows no symptoms. Initially a steady state viraemia occurs during the asymptomatic stage. This means that a dynamic equilibrium exists between the production and clearance of viral particles by the immune system. During the asymptomatic period up to a billion HIV particles and two billion CD4 cells are destroyed and produced each day. The CD4 count is initially normal and the viral load is low. Over time, the CD4 count will decline and the viral load will increase (see Figure 2.1 on page 26). This asymptomatic individual is still infectious and is able to transmit the virus.

Early symptomatic HIV infection

The immune system keeps the viral RNA at a constant level until viral replication becomes overwhelming. The CD4 count gradually declines over several years. The decline in CD4 count accelerates more rapidly one and a half to two years before an AIDS-defining illness starts (*Bartlett & Gallant 2000*).

Early symptomatic HIV infection is characterised by recurrent infections, bacterial pneumonia, pulmonary tuberculosis, herpes zoster infection, oral candidiasis and oral hairy leukoplakia.

Late stage HIV infection

Late stage disease is characterised by a CD4 count of less than 200 cells/µl, the development of opportunistic infections, selected tumours, muscle wasting and neurological complications – called AIDS. The median life expectancy of an untreated patient in the developed world once they have reached a CD4 count of less than 200 cells/µl is 3.7 years. The median CD4 count at the onset of the first AIDS-defining complication is 60–70 cells/µl. The median life expectancy in the developed world at this stage is slightly more than one year (*Bartlett & Gallant 2000*).

In the absence of any antiretroviral treatment the average duration from viral transmission to AIDS-defining diagnosis is ten years in the developed world and about eight years in the developing world (*Bartlett & Gallant 2000*).

Data from South Africa show that a patient with a median CD4 count of 111 cells/µl and extra-pulmonary TB has a median life expectancy of more than 24 months, while a patient with HIV wasting syndrome and a median CD4 count of 45 cells/µl has a median life expectancy of only one month. Life expectancy once AIDS-defining illnesses have started in countries like South Africa is generally lower than it is in the developed world. It is also apparent that the median CD4 count at which AIDS-defining illnesses start in developing countries is higher than that in the developed world (*Bartlett & Gallant 2002*).

Profiles of disease progression

Not everybody will progress from HIV infection to AIDS at the same rate.

Rapid progressors progress from HIV infection to AIDS within one or two years. These individuals may experience severe acute seroconversion disease and maintain a high set point viral load. They experience high levels of viral replication and a sharp drop in CD4 production. This drop in CD4 production prevents them from mounting an effective immune response and so they cannot control viral replication. Their high viral loads make them highly infectious.

The majority of HIV-infected individuals are intermediate progressors and are able to regulate viral replication. Over time, however, there is a steady decline in CD4 cells and eventual destruction of the immune system.

A small number of people are slow progressors or long-term non-progressors and are able to maintain very low viral load for a prolonged period of time without antiretroviral therapy. Some may even have undetectable viral loads and relatively high CD4 counts and a strong immune system. Many of these individuals have been infected for as long as 20 years without showing signs of progression.

Resistance to infection

There are some individuals who have remained HIV-negative in spite of repeated exposure to the virus. They include sex workers and some gay men.

CLINICAL STAGING

The World Health Organisation (WHO) has devised a clinical staging system, which is widely used in the developed world, but is dependent on CD4 counts so is difficult to use in the developing world. The system is used to define when a patient needs treatment to prevent opportunistic infections, when a patient has AIDS and when making treatment decisions. Refer to Table 2.1 for the WHO clinical staging system for adults (refer to Table 10.1 on page 151 for the WHO clinical staging system for children).

WHO clinical staging system for adults

Table 2.1	
Stage 1	
Seroconversion illness	
Asymptomatic infection	
Persistent generalised lymphadenopathy	
Performance status one *(fully active and asymptomatic)*	
Stage 2	
Less than 10% weight loss	
Herpes zoster infection	
Minor mucocutaneous manifestations	
Recurrent upper respiratory tract infections	
Performance status two *(symptomatic but nearly fully active)*	
Stage 3	
More than 10% weight loss	
Chronic diarrhoea for more than one month	
Prolonged fever	
Oral candida, chronic vaginal candidiasis	
Oral hairy leukoplakia	
Severe bacterial infections	
Pulmonary tuberculosis	
Performance status three *(in bed <50% of normal daytime)*	
Stage 4	
Extrapulmonary tuberculosis	
Pneumocystis pneumonia	
Cryptococcal meningitis	
Herpes simples virus ulcer >one month	
Oesophageal candidiasis	

Toxoplasmosis

Cryptosporidiosis

Isosporiasis

Cytomegalovirus

HIV wasting syndrome

HIV encephalopathy

Kaposi's sarcoma

Progressive multifocal leukoencephalopathy

Disseminated mycosis

Atypical mycobacteriosis

Non-typhoid *Salmonella* bacteraemia

Lymphoma

Recurrent pneumonia

Invasive cervical carcinoma

Performance status four *(confined to bed >50% of normal daytime)*

Source : Wilson et al. 2002

In South Africa and other African countries it is important to realise that patients may present differently from those in the developed world. For example, tuberculosis (TB) is the most common opportunistic infection complicating HIV and can occur at any stage of immunodeficiency. Early in HIV, TB presents in much the same way that it does in HIV-negative people. However, later in HIV, TB is often disseminated. Diarrhoeal disease and HIV wasting syndrome are also common in Africa.

CHAPTER 3

OPPORTUNISTIC INFECTIONS

Candice Bodkin

KEY CONCEPTS

- opportunistic infections
- immune system
- CD4 count
- viral load
- prevention and management
- tuberculosis

> HIV infection is the most potent risk factor for active tuberculosis and as a result TB has become the leading life-threatening opportunitic infection.
>
> *(Martinson et al. 2003)*

THE IMMUNE SYSTEM AND HIV AND AIDS

HIV and AIDS has the following effects on the immune system:

- It affects all aspects of the immune system.
- It reduces the effectiveness of cell-mediated immunity and humoral immunity.
- It reduces macrophage and monocyte function.
- It causes neutrophil dysregulation.

These effects on the immune system:

- reduce the body's ability to mount an immune response to a new antigen
- increase the risk of nosocomial infections
- increase the risk of resurgence of childhood infections in adulthood.

Why do HIV positive individuals get opportunistic infections?

Opportunistic infections arise because effective functioning of the immune system is reduced, predisposing the HIV-positive person to infections. Infections may be caused by organisms that are normally of low virulence or even organisms that are normally non-pathogenic. HIV-infected people are generally more prone to bacterial and fungal infections. HIV infection reduces immunity, predisposing the person to reactivation of endogenous infections such as tuberculosis (TB), toxoplasmosis, herpes, cryptosporidiosis, and cytomegalovirus. Infections may be atypical, in that they occur at unusual sites, have an unusual appearance and cause infection at multiple sites, or disseminated disease may occur. HIV-infected people are not only infected with opportunistic pathogens, but by normal pathogens as well.

CD4 count and opportunistic infection

Individuals with a CD4 count between 200–499 cells/µl are at an increased risk of *Mycobacterium* tuberculosis infection, oral candidiasis and herpes zoster infection. Once the CD4 count drops to 100–200 cells/µl the HIV-infected individual is at an increased risk of *Pneumocystis jiroveci*, oesophageal candidiasis and herpes simplex infection. Individuals with a CD4 count of less than 50 cells/µl are prone to *Toxoplasma gondii*, cytomegalovirus and progressive multifocal leukoencephalopathy (PML). However, it is important to realise that in South Africa, HIV-positive people may develop opportunistic infections at higher CD4 counts than infected people in the developed world. TB infection can occur at any stage of immunosuppression in Africa and is the most common opportunistic infection in southern Africa (*Cotton 2005*).

Prevalence of opportunistic pathogens

The pathogens that cause opportunistic infections vary, depending on the geographical location of the HIV-infected person. For example, *Mycobacterium tuberculosis* is more common as an opportunistic infection in sub-Saharan Africa than it is anywhere else in the world. Other opportunistic infections such as *Pneumocystis jiroveci* and cytomegalovirus will cause the same disease manifestation irrespective of geographical location (*Cotton 2005*).

COMMON OPPORTUNISTIC INFECTIONS

Oral infections

Oral manifestations occur in a large proportion of HIV-infected individuals. Oral manifestations of HIV are often missed, incorrectly diagnosed and inadequately managed. It is important to correctly diagnose and treat oral manifestations of HIV as these are uncomfortable for the patient. These diseases result in poor appetite and inability to eat which exacerbates weight loss in HIV and AIDS patients.

Candidiasis

Oral candidiasis presents as thick, white-creamy patches in the mouth, interspersed with red patches and accompanied by angular cheilitis. Oesophageal involvement is common. Oral candidiasis is treated with amphotericin B lozenges, oral nystatin suspension or oral fluconazole.

Oral hairy leukoplakia

Oral hairy leukoplakia is associated with the Epstein-Barr virus. It presents as white corrugated lesions on the lateral borders of the tongue. Oral hairy leukoplakia is usually painless and does not require treatment unless the patient requests it for cosmetic reasons. There has been a decrease in the incidence of this disease since the introduction of antiretroviral therapy (Reznik 2005).

Herpes simplex

Herpes simplex stomatitis is caused by herpes simplex viruses (HSV-1 and HSV-2). This viral infection is common and results in painful, recurrent oral ulcers, found generally on the lip as small crops of fluid-filled, painful vesicles. Over time, the vesicles rupture and form a small ulcer. The infection generally resolves on its own without treatment. In severe cases a topical antiviral may be applied (acyclovir).

Kaposi's sarcoma

Kaposi's sarcoma is the most frequent oral malignancy occurring in AIDS patients. The incidence has decreased since the introduction of antiretroviral therapy. The malignancy is associated with the Kaposi's sarcoma-associated herpes virus. Kaposi's sarcoma of the mouth can be macular, nodular, or raised and ulcerative (Reznik 2005). The colour of the lesion ranges from red to purple; the colour becomes darker as the lesion ages. Early malignancy may be asymptomatic, but as the malignancy progresses patients may have pain associated with ulceration, bleeding or superinfection. Treatment ranges from a local injection of chemotherapy to the surgical removal of the lesion. If the sarcoma has extended beyond the oral cavity, systemic chemotherapy may be required.

Periodontal disease

Periodontal disease presents as a red band along the gingival margin and may be accompanied by bleeding and discomfort. It is thought to be caused by a sub-gingival colonisation by *Candida albicans* (*Reznik 2005*). The patient should be referred to a dental professional for treatment. The nurse should encourage oral mouth rinsing with 0.12% chlorhexidine gluconate and good oral hygiene.

Aphthous ulcers

Aphthous ulcers occur on the buccal mucosa, on the floor of the mouth, ventral surface of the tongue, posterior oropharynx, and in the maxillary and mandibular vestibules. Lesions are characterised by a halo of inflammation, and a yellow-grey pseudomembranous covering. This ulcer can be very painful and can affect the person's ability to eat. In the immunocompromised HIV-infected individual these ulcers can last for more than 14 days. Treatment includes application of a topical corticosteroid and adequate pain control using paracetamol and topical 2% viscous lignocaine gel.

Skin infections

Herpes zoster

Shingles is caused by reactivation of Varicella-zoster virus and is known as herpes zoster infection. Shingles can be very painful and the pain can persist for weeks. Shingles is usually easy to identify as it presents as a unilateral, painful, vesicular, and erosive dermatological eruption (*Wilson et al. 2002*). The danger with shingles in AIDS patients is a secondary bacterial infection. Acyclovir, an antiviral used to treat shingles, may have to be accompanied by a topical/oral antibiotic and analgesia.

Molluscum contagiosum

The affected patient presents with 2–5 mm pearly flesh-coloured papules, often with a central umbilication. Molluscum contagiosum frequently occurs on the face, on the eyelids and in the anogenital region. Papules may number from one to many hundreds. Usually the infection is not treated, unless requested by the patient. Should the patient request it, a gentle application of liquid nitrogen may be used to remove papules. If the lesions are extensive, the patient should ideally be referred to a dermatologist. Complete eradication is difficult.

Kaposi's sarcoma

Kaposi's sarcoma is an endothelial cell tumour and may occur at any CD4 count but has a poorer prognosis if the CD4 count is very low. If Kaposi's sarcoma occurs on a mucocutaneous surface it merely poses a cosmetic problem and is not a serious threat to health, although cellulitis and infection are complications of mucocutaneous lesions. A lesion occurring in the gastrointestinal mucosa results in a chronic loss of blood as this surface is vascular. Kaposi's sarcoma may invade the viscera and lung parenchyma, and the lesions can bleed profusely. Visceral Kaposi's sarcoma may require systemic chemotherapy.

Scabies

Sarcoptes scabiei infection is particularly severe in immunocompromised individuals due to a very high mite population. Secondary staphylococcal infection is a risk. Treat scabies in an HIV-positive individual with 5% permethrin, 1% tindane or ivermectin 200–250 µg/kg.

Central nervous system infections

Cryptococcus neoformans

Cryptococcus neoformans is the most common cause of meningitis in HIV-infected individuals in Africa. The disease most commonly presents when the CD4 count drops below 100 cells/µl. The patient presents with meningo-encephalitis, severe headache, meningism and fever. Diagnosis of cryptococcal meningitis is made on lumber puncture. In the presence of *Cryptococcus neoformans* antigen the cerebrospinal fluid (CSF) will stain positive with India ink. *Cryptococcus neoformans* can also be cultured from CSF and from blood. Treat cryptococcal meningitis with amphotericin B for two weeks. Following cryptococcal infection, lifelong prophylaxis with fluconazole is recommended.

Poor prognostic features include:

- comatose or confused patient
- hypoglycaemia (<2.0 g/dl glucose)
- CD4 count of <50 cells/µl
- blindness
- cranial nerve palsies
- comorbid disease.

Mycobacteria tuberculosis

Mycobacteria tuberculosis meningitis can be a severe and life-threatening condition and is a common opportunistic infection in HIV-positive people in southern Africa. It can occur at any stage of HIV infection and is not confined to those with a very low CD4 count. *Mycobacteria tuberculosis* is treated with TB treatment regimen 1 for nine months (refer to the discussion of TB on pages 43–46 for the full drug regimen). Decadron can be added if signs and symptoms of raised intracranial pressure are observed.

Bacterial meningitis

Bacterial meningitis is suspected in an HIV-positive patient presenting with severe headache, neck stiffness, photophobia, fever, vomiting, altered level of consciousness, focal signs and seizures. Lumbar puncture is necessary to diagnose bacterial meningitis.

The following organisms cause bacterial meningitis in HIV-positive individuals:

* *Streptococcus pneumoniae*
* *Listeria monocytogenes*
* *Haemophilus influenzae.*

Treatment depends on the causative organism. If the HIV-positive patient has meningococcal meningitis the patient should be isolated for 48 hours following the start of treatment. The patient's contacts should take ciprofloxacin 500 mg PO as post-exposure prophylaxis as soon as possible after the patient's diagnosis.

Toxoplasmosis

The seroprevalence of *Toxoplasma gondii* in South Africa is 20%. Most clinical disease is due to reactivation of existing disease. Toxoplasmosis manifests as encephalitis in AIDS patients, who present with confusion, lethargy, low grade fever, weakness, ataxia, apraxia, seizures and sensory loss. Presumptive diagnosis is made on the triad of positive *Toxoplasma* serology, characteristic radiographs and a positive response to empiric anti-*Toxoplasma* therapy. The standard treatment is with co-trimoxazole for four weeks. Patients who cannot tolerate co-trimoxazole can be treated with clindamycin.

Cytomegalovirus

Most AIDS patients infected with cytomegalovirus (CMV) develop retinitis. Cytomegalovirus causes gastrointestinal infection in a small proportion of AIDS patients infected with the virus.

CMV retinitis causes progressive visual deterioration, until ultimately the patient becomes blind. Initially the patient will be asymptomatic but as the disease progresses the patient may complain of floaters and reduced visual acuity. As the retinitis is a necrotic process, antiviral treatment can cause atrophic regression of the necrotic lesion, but this necrotic lesion will never regain function.

Diagnosis is made using visual inspection by ophthalmoscopy carried out by an experienced doctor. Treatment is with intravitreal ganciclovir, which should be started by an experienced ophthalmologist and is used according to the following criteria:

- the patient should have visual acuity of 60/60 or better
- there should be no CMV retinitis in the macula
- there should be no optic nerve involvement.

Complicating infections should be treated.

Peripheral neuropathy

Peripheral neuropathy, mainly affecting the feet, may be the result of antiretroviral therapy, or may be due to the HIV disease process itself. It occurs in about one third of patients with a CD4 count of less than 200 cells/μl. There are reversible factors such as alcohol, vitamin deficiencies and drugs that can exacerbate the neuropathy and patients should be strongly counselled against alcohol use. Presentation can vary from mild numbness and 'pins and needles' to debilitating pain. If the peripheral neuropathy is the result of antiretroviral drug toxicity the offending drug should be changed. If the peripheral neuropathy is due to the HIV disease process, supportive treatment is offered. This includes the administration of nonsteroidal anti-inflammatory agents. Thiamine is also used, and patients taking isoniazid should be given pyridoxine. Other agents useful in pain syndromes include amitriptyline or carbamazepine. Where the pain is refractory to treatment, give a long-acting narcotic.

AIDS-related dementia

Initially the presentation of AIDS dementia is subtle – the patient may complain of short-term memory loss and difficulty concentrating. Some patients may present with depression, others with unexplained seizures or psychomotor retardation. An MRI scan shows diffuse cortical loss. The only treatment for AIDS dementia is antiretroviral therapy, which should include zidovudine if possible. The response to antiretrovirals can be impressive.

Neurosyphilis

Neurosyphilis is more common in HIV-infected individuals than in others infected with syphilis. Neurosyphilis in HIV-positive individuals may have the following presentation:

- meningovascular syphilis
- tabes dorsalis
- general paresis of the insane.

Meningovascular syphilis presents as a low-grade meningitis with headaches, irritability, cranial nerve palsies and pupillary abnormalities. Some patients may even present with a cerebrovascular accident.

The posterior spinal column is involved in tabes dorsalis. The patient presents with impaired proprioception and reduced tendon reflexes. The patient may report 'lightning' or 'stabbing' pains in their legs.

The patient with general paresis of the insane presents with subtle changes in their personality, forgetfulness, irritability and lack of concentration. As the disease progresses the patient presents with delusions of grandeur, manic symptoms and/or dementia. Examination reveals tremors of the tongue, lips and hands. Incontinence may develop at a late stage.

Neurosyphilis is treated with aqueous procaine penicillin G 2.4 MU IMI daily plus probenicid 500 mg QID for ten days; followed by benzathine penicillin weekly for three weeks.

Gastrointestinal infection

Diarrhoea

Between 40% and 90% of HIV-positive patients will present with diarrhoea at some stage of their illness. How the diarrhoea is treated and managed depends on the degree of immune suppression and the type of diarrhoeal illness.

Acute diarrhoea

Acute diarrhoea is defined as diarrhoea consisting of four watery stools per day lasting more than one week but less than one month.

Typical causative organisms in HIV-positive patients include:

- *Campylobacter jejuni*
- Listeria
- *Clostridium difficile*
- Shigella.

Criteria for hospital admission include:

- severe dehydration with circulatory collapse
- blood pressure <80/60 mmhg
- confusion
- fever with a temperature of >39 °C
- the patient needing intravenous fluids and antibiotics.

Treatment includes replacement of fluids, correction of electrolytes and dietary modification. Empiric antibiotic treatment includes amoxicillin 500 mg TDS PO or co-trimoxazole two tablets BD PO for seven days. Antidiarrhoeal agents should only be used if acute infective colitis has been excluded. It can include loperamide and codeine phosphate. The patient should be advised to limit their intake of caffeine, milk and milk products.

Chronic diarrhoea

Chronic diarrhoea is defined as three or more loose stools per day for more than 30 days. Common causative organisms:

- Protozoa (microsporidia, *Cryptosporidia, Isospora belli*)
- Mycobacteria
- Viruses (CMV)

Admission criteria are the same as those for acute diarrhoea.

Treatment includes replacement of fluids, correction of electrolytes and dietary modification. Antibiotic treatment depends on the causative organism.

Salmonella septicaemia

Non-typhoid salmonella species acquired from contaminated food can cause severe recurrent septicaemia in AIDS patients. Salmonella septicaemia presents with high fever and septicaemia and is rapidly fatal if not treated promptly. Diarrhoea is often absent. This infection can be prevented by cooking food, washing fruit and vegetables thoroughly, and avoiding unpasteurised milk.

Treatment includes aggressive volume replacement therapy. Patients are treated with a third-generation cephalosporin or quinolone IV and are given four to six weeks of oral therapy to prevent relapse.

Oesophageal candidiasis

Oesophageal candidiasis in HIV-positive individuals commonly presents with odynophagia and dysphagia. These patients may also present with wasting and dehydration because they cannot eat or drink.

Treatment includes rehydration. If electrolyte imbalances are present, these should be corrected. Fluconazole 200 mg daily for 14 days is the recommended treatment. Fluconazole may be administered intravenously if it cannot be tolerated orally.

Cryptosporidiosis

Cryptosporidiosis is caused by enteric protozoa that cause severe diarrhoea and weight loss in patients with AIDS. Currently there is no effective treatment, so care is supportive. Highly active antiretroviral therapy at optimum dosages may resolve the infection.

Mycobacterium avium

Mycobacterium avium is an end-stage AIDS disease and occurs when the CD4 count is extremely low. The presentation of *Mycobacterium avium* is non-specific. Patients may present with fever, weight loss, diarrhoea, anaemia, abdominal discomfort due to hepatosplenomegaly and intra-abdominal lymphadenopathy.

Diagnosis is made on a positive mycobacterial blood culture. *Mycobacterium avium* is treated with a combination of antimicrobial agents (clarithromycin and ethambutol).

Pulmonary infections

Community-acquired pneumonia

Community-acquired pneumonia in HIV-positive individuals may be caused by the following organisms:

- *Streptococcus pneumoniae*
- *Haemophilus influenzae*.

Community-acquired pneumonia can occur in all HIV-positive individuals at any stage of HIV infection. Other risk factors for community-acquired pneumonia in HIV-positive individuals include:

- smoking
- drug abuse
- neutropenia
- hypoalbuminaemia.

The hospital admission criteria for HIV-positive patients with community-acquired pneumonia include:

- temperature >39 °C
- blood pressure <100/60 mmhg
- respiratory rate >30 breaths per minute
- dehydration
- cyanosis
- age >60 years
- multi-lobar pneumonia
- confusion
- co-morbid disease.

The following investigations are required:

- blood cultures
- sputum for acid-fast bacillus, gram stain, and MC&S
- chest X-ray.

Treatment is usually supportive. A second generation cephalosporin can be prescribed for seven days. The patient may require broader gram-negative cover, depending on the blood culture results.

Pneumocystis jiroveci

Pneumocystis pneumonia can be difficult to diagnose and requires a high index of clinical suspicion. The diagnostic triad of fever, exertional dyspnoea and non-productive cough only occurs in 50% of patients.

Almost all patients with pneumocystis pneumonia have at least two of the following symptoms:

- fever
- cough
- dyspnoea
- elevated lactate dehydrogenase
- PaO_2 <75 mmhg

Careful history taking may reveal long-standing dyspnoea over a period of weeks to months. Fine crackles may be heard on auscultation of the chest. A chest X-ray may reveal diffuse interstitial or perihilar infiltrates, but a wide variety of chest X-ray abnormalities are possible and it may appear normal in mild disease.

Pneumocystis pneumonia may be confused with many other respiratory diseases such as tuberculosis, or a respiratory tract infection due to a viral, bacterial or fungal infection.

Treatment is with co-trimoxazole and should be continued for at least 21 days. Start prophylaxis after treatment. Prophylaxis for pneumocystis pneumonia is also needed by HIV-positive patients with a CD4 count of less than 200 cells/μl, irrespective of whether or not they have had a previous pneumocystis infection.

Other conditions

Lymphoma

Several different types of lymphoma occur at increased frequency in HIV-positive individuals. Lymphoma may occur at any CD4 count but the prognosis is worse if the CD4 count is low. Typical lymphomas occurring with increased frequency in HIV infection include: Hodgkin's disease, immunoblastic lymphoma, Burkitt's lymphoma, and non-Hodgkin's B cell lymphoma. HIV-positive patients are more likely to present with extranodal lymphoma and non-Hodgkin's lymphoma at usual sites. Lymphomas are treated with chemotherapy, but HIV-positive individuals may require lower doses due to bone marrow fragility.

HIV wasting

HIV wasting is one of the hallmark symptoms of AIDS. HIV wasting can be defined as weight loss that exceeds 10% of the patient's baseline weight plus either chronic diarrhoea or fever, for more than 30 days, without any concurrent illness. The patient presents with a loss of muscle mass, particularly in the temporal region, and complains of generalised fatigue and weakness. HIV-related wasting and its management are discussed in detail in Chapter 5.

TUBERCULOSIS

The dramatic spread of HIV through sub-Saharan Africa has been accompanied by a four-fold increase in TB prevalence. Around 50% of new adult cases of TB in South Africa are co-infected with HIV. HIV-positive individuals have a six-fold greater risk of tuberculosis (TB) infection compared with HIV-negative individuals. Antiretroviral therapy has been found to reduce the risk of TB among HIV-positive individuals. Active TB may arise as a result of reactivation, rapid progression of a primary infection or re-infection from outside. TB often arises before other opportunistic infections arise, probably because *Mycobacterium tuberculosis* is a more virulent organism than most of the organisms that cause opportunistic infections.

The incidence of TB increases initially after the initiation of antiretroviral therapy, particularly in individuals with a CD4 count of less than 50 cells/µl. This increase in TB infection is due to active undiagnosed TB being unmasked by the immune reconstitution that follows the initiation of antiretroviral therapy. After the initial increase in tuberculosis, the incidence of TB decreases by 59% in individuals on antiretroviral therapy. However, the TB infection rates of individuals on antiretroviral therapy remains high (12%) (*Churchyard & Metcalf 2005*).

Diagnosis of tuberculosis

Typical signs and symptoms of tuberculosis include:

* cough lasting more than two weeks
* fever lasting more than two weeks
* night sweats
* other symptoms such as pleuritic chest pain and haemoptyses
* weight loss of more than 1.5 kg in the past four weeks.

Patients with one or more signs of tuberculosis should be investigated further for TB:

* Collect two early morning sputum samples for acid-fast bacillus (AFB) staining
* The diagnosis of TB can be made if one or more specimens is positive for AFBs.

The following HIV-positive patients presenting with tuberculosis should be admitted:

* very ill patient
* fever of more than 40 °C
* significant haemoptyses
* co-morbid disease that is poorly controlled: diabetes, epilepsy, congestive cardiac failure, alcoholism, or another AIDS-defining condition.

Treatment of tuberculosis

Regimen 1: New adults (>50 kg)

2 month initial phase

Combination tablet (RHZE) 120/60/300/200 mg x 5 tablets (rifampicin, isoniazid, pyrazinamide, ethambutol) given Monday to Friday

4 month continuation phase

Combination tablet (RH) 300/150 mg x 2 tablets (rifampicin and isoniazid) given Monday to Friday

---

Regimen 2: Retreatment of adults (>50 kg)

2 month initial phase

Combination tablet (RHZE) 120/60/300/200 mg x 5 tablets (rifampicin, isoniazid, pyrazinamide, ethambutol) + streptomycin* 750 mg IMI given Monday to Friday

3rd month

Combination tablet (RHZE) 120/60/300/200 mg x 5 tablets (rifampicin, isoniazid, pyrazinamide, ethambutol) given Monday to Friday

5 month continuation phase

Combination tablet (RH) 150/100 mg x 3 tablets (rifampicin and isoniazid) + ethambutol 400 mg (2 tablets) given Monday to Friday

* don't give streptomycin to patients older than 65 years

Source: Department of Health 2004. National Antiretroviral Treatment Guidelines. Pretoria: Department of Health

Management of concomitant tuberculosis and HIV in adults

If tuberculosis is diagnosed in an HIV-positive individual there are two possible treatment scenarios to consider. Refer to Chapter 10 for the management of tuberculosis in children.

The patient develops tuberculosis whilst on antiretroviral therapy

Antiretroviral therapy should be continued throughout TB treatment. However changes to the antiretroviral regimen will have to be instituted.

HIV-positive patients on first-line HIV treatment regimen

- If the patient is on nevirapine, the nevirapine should be changed to efavirenz. If efavirenz cannot be tolerated by the patient, the patient may continue taking nevirapine, under the guidance of an HIV specialist. These patients require monthly liver enzyme monitoring.

HIV patients on second-line HIV treatment regimen

- The lopinavir/ritonavir dose should be altered to 400/400 mg every 12 hours. This implies that the patient should take three extra capsules of ritonavir. This treatment regimen should continue for at least three weeks after the completion of anti-TB treatment.

Patient presents with tuberculosis before commencing antiretroviral therapy

- If the patient has no history of a WHO stage IV condition and their CD4 count is greater than 200 cells/μl, antiretroviral therapy is not indicated. The patient may be started on tuberculosis treatment. The patient should be reassessed for antiretroviral therapy after the completion of anti-TB treatment.
- If the patient has a WHO stage IV condition and/or has a CD4 count of less than 200 cells/μl, then TB treatment should be started and antiretroviral therapy should be started two months after the start of TB treatment.
- If the patient has a CD4 count of less than 50cells/μl and has tuberculosis, then anti-TB treatment should be started as soon as possible. If after two weeks the patient is tolerating the TB treatment then antiretroviral therapy may be started.

Shared side effects of tuberculosis treatment and antiretroviral therapy

Concomitant anti-tuberculosis treatment and antiretroviral therapy has the following shared side effects: nausea, hepatitis, peripheral neuropathy and rash.

TB/HIV treatment and DOTS

DOTS is directly observed tuberculosis treatment short-course. Integrating TB and HIV treatment in rural, resources-limited settings using the existing TB DOTS infrastructure has been shown to be feasible, safe and effective.

CHAPTER 4

PRINCIPLES OF ANTIRETROVIRAL THERAPY

Candice Bodkin

> The advent of highly active antiretroviral therapy has revolutionised the treatment of HIV, with both patients and physicians enjoying the resultant increases in both quality and quantity of life
>
> *(Jones and Nelson 2005)*

INTRODUCTION

The introduction of antiretroviral therapy has led to a reduction in the progression of HIV to AIDS and has resulted in the reduction of AIDS-related deaths. However, despite the introduction of antiretroviral therapy, HIV and AIDS-infected individuals remain at risk of opportunistic infections and HIV-related tumours, but the risk is considerably lower than those who are not on such treatment. Treatment failure can be due to factors related to the HI virus, the drugs and to the individual on therapy. Adherence to therapy is particularly important. If a person regularly misses more than one dose every ten days, using twice daily therapy, he or she is at a substantially increased risk of treatment failure. Before starting antiretroviral therapy take a comprehensive patient history and make a thorough patient assessment.

HISTORY TAKING AND ASSESSMENT

History

It is important to take a clear and accurate history at the patient's initial presentation for HIV care. A patient presenting at an HIV facility for the first time is likely to be anxious. HIV-positive patients should be approached with empathy, sensitivity and with a non-judgemental attitude. Good communication skills are important to ensure that a trusting relationship is established.

The history should include the following:

Sociodemographic details

* record the patient's name and surname
* age and birth date
* occupation
* marital status.

The main complaint

Record in the patient's own words the reason for attending the HIV clinic. With respect to the main complaint establish the following:

* its severity
* its duration
* its associated features
* its provoking factors
* its alleviating factors.

History of HIV diagnosis

Establish where and when the patient first found out that they are HIV-positive. It is important to determine whether the HIV test conducted was sensitive and specific. In addition, it is important to work out approximately how long the patient has been HIV-positive. This may be calculated from the time of the positive test. If the patient initally tested negative and then tested positive at a recent second test, you can assume that the patient seroconverted recently.

Medical history

Many medical conditions can affect the choice of antiretroviral therapy. Ask about the following medical conditions:

- hypertension
- type 1 and type 2 diabetes
- cardiovascular disease
- hepatic and renal disease
- previous or current malignant conditions
- haematological conditions
- other medical conditions.

Sexually transmitted infections (STIs) include syphilis, gonorrhoea, herpes simplex, pelvic inflammatory disease, and anogenital warts. The patient should be questioned about exposure to tuberculosis, any previous history of tuberculosis and any previous treatment of tuberculosis. Ask about hepatitis A, B or C, pneumococcal infection, influenza, and varicella zoster. Ask about recent or past influenza and pneumococcal vaccination.

Question the patient about the following HIV-related signs and symptoms:

- weight loss
- night sweats
- muscle weakness
- chronic cough
- chronic diarrhoea
- peripheral neuropathy
- severe headache
- difficulty swallowing.

Mental health history

The stigma and isolation associated with an HIV-positive diagnosis may result in depression, anxiety, insomnia and social withdrawal. Furthermore, advanced HIV infection may cause dementia.

Family history

- Determine the age, health status, medical history of the patient's parents, siblings and children. Extended family members may be included if their medical history is significant. If a family member has died, attempt to determine the cause of death.

- Determine whether any other family members are HIV-positive.
- Ask specifically about family history related to cardiovascular disease, tuberculosis, and diabetes mellitus.

Medication history

It is important to know what treatment the patient has already received for their HIV infection, particularly any antiretroviral therapy. If the patient was on antiretroviral therapy establish which regimen the patient was on, whether or not they developed adverse reactions, whether or not they were adherent and their reasons for stopping treatment if they did so.

Ask about previous and current medication. Attempt to name the drugs and include dosages. Include any history of herbal remedies, traditional medicines, over-the-counter medication and alternative and complementary medicine. Establish whether the patient has allergies to any medication.

Social history

This should include:

- place of birth
- highest level of education
- type of occupation and details about occupation
- current place of residence and with whom
- childcare responsibilities
- history of domestic violence
- pets (risk of toxoplasmosis)
- alcohol use, cigarette smoking or use of other drugs
- social support network
- travel history.

When taking the social history establish whether or not the HIV-infected individual is using condoms. Establish whether a woman is using any other form of contraception. Determine the type of contraception and how consistently it is used. It may be necessary at this point to determine the number of sexual partners.

Assessment

Investigations

The following screening tests are recommended:

- The *full blood count (FBC)* is used to detect anaemia, leucopenia, lymphopenia and thrombocytopenia. The result of the FBC will influence decisions made about the treatment regimen and choice of antiretroviral.

- *Urea and electrolytes (U & E) and liver function tests* are used to measure kidney and liver function. Liver function is particularly important when deciding upon an antiretroviral regimen and for monitoring a patient on antiretroviral therapy.

- A *chest X-ray* will assist in diagnosis of tuberculosis and serves as a baseline for patients who are at high risk for pulmonary disease.

- If tuberculosis is suspected, early morning sputum samples should be sent for an *acid-fast bacillus (AFB)* test. Tuberculin (PPD) skin testing may be required to detect tuberculosis.

- *PAP smear* and gynaecological evaluation serves as a baseline for the detection of the development of any gynaecological cancers or disease.

- *CD4 cell count* is a standard test to stage the disease and make therapeutic decisions regarding antiretroviral treatment and other prophylactic treatment.

- A *viral load* is necessary as a baseline and to measure viral response to antiretroviral therapy.

- *Serology for hepatitis B and hepatitis C and serology for Toxoplasmosis and Cytomegalovirus* are useful tests. Vaccination against Hepatitis B can be offered.

Physical examination

The physical examination must be conducted in a private place. Ask the patient to undress for the physical exam. Provide the patient with a gown and allow him or her to lie on a bed covered with a sheet/blanket.

General

- Assess vital signs (blood pressure, pulse, respiration rate and temperature).

- The general examination should include: cyanosis, pallor, jugular venous pressure, clubbing, oedema, lymphadenopathy and hydration status.

- The patient should ideally be weighed and their height measured.
- Check for evidence of wasting and lipodystrophy.

Eyes
- Examine the conjunctiva for abnormalities.
- Fundoscopy can be conducted:
    - Look for 'cotton wool' spots due to occlusion of retinal capillaries.
    - Look for infiltrates and haemorrhages caused by CMV retinitis.

Oropharynx
Look for:
- oral candidiasis
- oral hairy leukoplakia
- purple spots of Kaposi's sarcoma.

Lymph nodes
Look for:
- generalised lymphadenopathy
- regional lymphadenopathy may be associated with localised pathology (TB or lymphoma).

Lungs
- Inspect, percuss, palpate and auscultate.

Liver and spleen
- Determine whether the liver and/or spleen are enlarged.
- Organomegaly typically reflects disseminated infection with tuberculosis or histoplasmosis; it may also be a sign of lymphoma.

Pelvic exam
- Observe the external genitalia for ulcers, lesions or abnormal discharge.

Neurological
- Motor deficits may reflect space-occupying lesions in the central nervous system (toxoplasmosis, lymphoma, progressive multifocal leukoencephalopathy, neurosyphilis).
- Assess for peripheral neuropathy.
- Assess for reduced short-term memory, reduced concentration and sensorimotor retardation (AIDS dementia).

Skin

Assess for:

- pruritic papular lesions (bacterial folliculitis and scabies)
- pearly papules, with central umbilication (*Molluscum contagiosum*)
- painful vesicular rash (herpes simplex virus)
- shingles (varicella zoster)
- scaly, erythematous areas on the face (seborrhoeic dermatitis)
- purplish macules or plaques (Kaposi's sarcoma).

GOALS OF ANTIRETROVIRAL THERAPY

Goals of antiretroviral therapy include (*Bartlett & Gallant 2000*):

- Clinical goals:
  Prolong life and improve the quality of life.
- Virologic goals:
  Reduce the viral load, halt disease progression and prevent or reduce resistant variants.
- Immunologic goals:
  Achieve immune reconstitution that is quantitative (CD4 count in normal range) and qualitative (pathogen-specific immune response).
- Therapeutic goals:
  The antiretroviral therapy should achieve therapeutic goals, have few side effects and be realistic in terms of compliance.
- Epidemiological goals:
  Reduce HIV transmission.

Antiretroviral therapy reduces viral load initially, however, it does not offer a cure for HIV and AIDS infection. Virtually all studies show viral rebound within 12 weeks of discontinuing antiretroviral therapy (*Bartlett & Gallant 2000*).

WHEN SHOULD ANTIRETROVIRAL THERAPY BE STARTED?

The following individuals should receive antiretroviral therapy (Department of Health (DOH) 2004):

- CD4 count of <200 cells/μl irrespective of WHO stage
  OR
- WHO stage 4 disease irrespective of CD4 count

• Antiretroviral treatment should not be started if it is unlikely that the patient will be adherent, which suggests that they are not psychologically ready for treatment. There are certain psycho-social factors that suggest that a patient is more likely to be adherent to treatment, but there are no absolute predictors for reduced adherence. Adherence and the factors influencing it are discussed in detail later in the chapter.

Relative merits of early and delayed treatment (*Bartlett & Gallant 2000*)

Early Treatment	Delayed Treatment
Control viral replication	Poor quality of life with treatment
Prevent progressive immune deficiency	Earlier drug resistance
Delay progression to AIDS and death	Limited future drug options
Prevent resistance when fully effective	Long-term drug toxicity
Better tolerability of drugs	Duration of effectiveness is unknown
Reduce viral transmission	Risk of transmission of resistant strains

Table 4.1

In South Africa it is generally accepted that a patient should not start treatment too early in the course of infection because this would need excellent adherence for many years, with little health benefits for the patient. In addition, early use of antiretroviral therapy increases the chance of drug toxicity, and increases the chance of drug resistance, which would then require more complex and potentially toxic therapies once the patient has developed symptoms. A resistant virus in a relatively well patient is also more likely to be transmitted to sexual partners.

ANTIRETROVIRAL THERAPY

Antiretroviral therapy can be divided into three main classes:
• Nucleoside and nucleotide reverse transcriptase inhibitors (NRTIs)
• Non-nucleoside reverse transcriptase inhibitors (NNRTIs)
• Protease inhibitors (PIs)

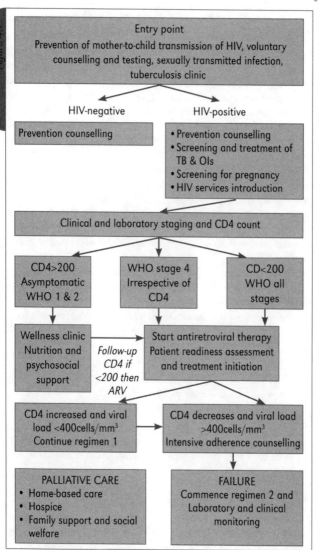

Algorithm for the management of HIV-positive adults

Source: Department of Health 2004. National Antiretroviral Treatment Guidelines. Pretoria: Department of Health.

NUCLEOSIDE AND NUCLEOTIDE REVERSE TRANSCRIPTASE INHIBITORS (NRTIs)

Nucleoside and nucleotide reverse transcriptase inhibitors are synthetic analogues of naturally occurring nucleosides that are used by cells for DNA replication. NRTIs act as false substrates for the viral enzyme reverse transcriptase and stop the process of transcription and prevents the virus from completing the process of transcribing its viral RNA into viral DNA.

In general, NRTIs have good bio-availability and can be taken with or without food. Didanosine is the exception; this drug should preferably be given without food.

As the NRTIs have limited plasma binding they are distributed fairly widely throughout the body. These drugs can be found in most tissues, in cerebrospinal fluid, in the placenta, and in breast milk.

The NRTIs are not metabolised by the P450 system. The advantage of this is that drug interactions occurring via the P450 system, such as is found in certain anti-tuberculous drugs, are unlikely. The NRTIs are mostly excreted via the renal system.

NRTIs prescribed in South Africa include, zidovudine, didanosine, stavudine, lamivudine and abacavir. All are available in liquid formulation for paediatric use.

The nucleotide RTI, tenofovir, should soon be registered for use in South Africa.

Zidovudine

Zidovudine (ZDV or AZT) was the first registered antiretroviral agent. Zidovudine is a thymidine analogue (*Patel et al. 2005*).

Lamivudine

Lamivudine is a cytidine analogue. Lamivudine is used widely in adults and in children as it is one of the most well-tolerated nucleoside reverse transcriptase inhibitors (*Patel et al. 2005*).

Stavudine

Stavudine is a thymidine analogue. Zidovudine is also a thymidine analogue and the co-administration of stavudine and AZT is not recommended. Stavudine should also not be taken concurrently with didanosine due to overlapping toxicity (*Patel et al. 2005*).

Didanosine

Didanosine has a long half-life and can thus be administered as a once daily dose. Didanosine is rapidly degraded in an acidic media and thus requires buffering by an antacid for optimal absorption. It is for this reason that didanosine is given separately from food.

NON-NUCLEOSIDE REVERSE TRANSCRIPTASE INHIBITORS (NNRTIs)

The non-nucleoside reverse transcriptase inhibitors directly inhibit the action of the enzyme reverse transcriptase. They can therefore effectively suppress HIV replication. However, the entire class of NNRTIs can be rendered ineffective by a single mutation in the reverse transcriptase gene. This means that high-level resistance can develop rapidly and they must always be used in combination with other drugs, usually with two NRTIs. This class of drugs also causes hepatotoxicity so the patient's liver function should be monitored.

NNRTIs available in South Africa include:

Nevirapine

Nevirapine is used extensively in neonates and in children. Nevirapine is also the drug of choice for the prevention of mother-to-child transmission (PMTCT) of HIV. For PMTCT a single 200 mg tablet is administered to the woman at the onset of labour. Nevirapine is also given to the neonate; 0.2 mg/kg is administered within 72 hours of birth.

Nevirapine is widely distributed in the tissues and can cross the placenta. Nevirapine has a long half-life and HIV-suppressive concentrations can be maintained for up to two weeks following a single dose.

However, nevirapine can cause potentially fatal hepatotoxicity and severe hypersensitivity reactions. Hepatotoxicity is more likely to occur within the first few months of treatment. It is for this reason that liver enzymes require close monitoring. During pregnancy nevirapine replaces efavirenz due to the potentially teratogenic effects of efavirenz. However, the pregnant woman has an increased risk of developing hepatotoxicity.

Nevirapine can also cause a severe, life-threatening skin reaction. Like hepatotoxicity, the skin reaction is more likely to occur in the early months of nevirapine administration. Cases of Stevens-Johnson syndrome and epidermal necrolyis have been reported (Patel et al. 2005).

Efavirenz

Efavirenz has been included in the first line antiretroviral regimen in South Africa and is used extensively in children over the age of three and in adults.

It can cause central nervous system side effects. In pregnancy, efavirenz can be replaced with nevirapine.

PROTEASE INHIBITORS (PIs)

Protease inhibitors block the HIV protease enzyme. This prevents maturation of viral particles. PIs can also cause potent suppression of viral replication. However, they must always be used in combination and are usually reserved for second-line therapy if the intial treatment regimen of two NRTIs plus one NNRTI fails. They have many side effects, particularly gastrointestinal, which reduce tolerability, adherence and absorption. Furthermore, PIs cause glucose intolerance, insulin resistance, hyperlipidaemia and lipodystrophy.

PIs available in South Africa include:

- indinavir
- ritonavir
- lopinavir-ritonavir – a PI co-formulation.

CLINICAL GUIDELINES FOR ANTIRETROVIRAL THERAPY IN ADULTS, MARCH 2005

South Africa has produced local clinical guidelines for antiretroviral therapy in adults. The guidelines provide three regimens. *(Source: The International Association of Physicians in AIDS Care and the Southern African HIV/AIDS Clinicians Society found at www.iapac.org)*

First-line antiretroviral regimen (Regimen 1)

> Stavudine 40 mg BD + Lamivudine 150 mg BD + Efavirenz 600 mg

The first-line antiretroviral regimen is prescribed when an HIV-positive patient presents at the antiretroviral clinic for the first time. This patient is generally healthy. This implies that they have no hepatic or renal conditions or any other major medical problems. Prior to starting antiretroviral therapy the patient should meet the inclusion criteria. This means that they must have a CD4 count of less than 200 cells/μl or they must present with a Stage 4 AIDS-defining condition.

This first-line regimen should not be given to pregnant women as efavirenz is teratogenic. If this regimen is prescribed to a woman of child-bearing age a reliable form of contraception should be offered.

Furthermore, as efavirenz has central nervous system side effects, this regimen should not be offered to any patient with a serious psychiatric disorder.

Major potential toxicities

Stavudine (d4T) can cause peripheral neuropathy, which can be exacerbated by the concomitant use of tuberculosis treatment. Stavudine also causes lipodystrophic changes, which are changes in body fat distribution. Pancreatitis is a serious adverse reaction to stavudine and should be ruled out if the patient presents with abdominal pain. Another serious adverse reaction to stavudine is lactic acidosis. Lactic acidosis should be considered if the patient presents with nausea, vomiting and abdominal pain, dyspnoea and fatigue and weight loss.

Efavirenz should be avoided in individuals with psychiatric illness as it may cause confusion and psychosis. Even individuals without psychiatric illness may experience central nervous system effects. It is for this reason that efavirenz is preferably given at night. Efavirenz is also toxic to the liver and liver enzymes must be closely monitored. Liver toxicity should be suspected in a patient presenting with jaundice and liver tenderness. A severe rash is a potentially serious side effect of NNRTIs. Patients on NNRTIs should be warned of this and should be advised to report to their healthcare provider as soon as possible if they develop any rash.

Potential side effects of the first-line regimen (Regimen 1)

The following are potential side effects of the first-line regimen (Regimen 1):

Somnolence	Dizziness	Fatigue
Insomnia	Nausea	Diarrhoea
Abdominal pain	Confusion	Headache
Mild rash	Nightmares	

First-line antiretroviral regimen (Regimen 1b)

Stavudine 40 mg BD + Lamivudine 150 mg BD + Nevirapine 200 mg BD

The first-line antiretroviral regimen (1b) is the preferred first-line regimen for pregnant women, because the teratogenic efavirenz is replaced with nevirapine. Nevirapine, also a NNRTI, has two serious side effects: hepatoxicity and a skin rash. Pregnant women starting antiretroviral therapy for the first time should start with nevirapine 200 mg once daily for two weeks. If they tolerate the nevirapine 200 mg once daily then the dose may be increased to 200 mg twice daily. The other two drugs should be started at the same time as the nevirapine at their recommended dosages. As pregnant women have an increased risk of developing hepatotoxicity due to nevirapine, their liver enzymes should be checked at least every two weeks for the first few weeks of treatment.

The first-line antiretroviral regimen (Regimen 1b) has drug interactions with tuberculosis treatment. If the patient requires TB treatment while on this regimen, the nevirapine should be replaced with efavirenz. Nevirapine may only be continued during TB treatment in a select few cases, and then monthly liver enzyme monitoring is required.

Major potential toxicities

Nevirapine is hepatotoxic. Patients presenting with jaundice, abdominal pain and liver tenderness should be investigated for hepatotoxicity. Nevirapine can also cause a severe skin rash and Stevens-Johnson syndrome.

Potential side effects of the first-line regimen (Regimen 1b)

The following are potential side effects of the first-line regimen (Regimen 1b):

Insomnia	Headache	Mild rash
Nausea	Fatigue	Fever
Diarrhoea	Abdominal discomfort	

Second-line antiretroviral regimen (Regimen 2)

Zidovudine 300 mg BD + Didanosine 200 mg daily + Lopinavir/ritonavir 400 mg/100 mg BD

The second-line regimen is prescribed for patients who:
- have had antiretroviral therapy before, and were not adherent
- have developed serious adverse reactions on the first-line regimens
- have developed drug resistance to the first-line regimens
- had drug interactions while on the first-line regimens.

The second-line regimen can be used by patients on TB treatment. However, the dosages must be adjusted. If the patient is on TB treatment the lopinavir/

ritonavir combination will have to be increased from 400/100 mg BD to 400/400 mg BD. The extra ritonavir may be discontinued two weeks after completing TB treatment.

Major potential toxicities

Zidovudine (AZT) can cause severe anaemia and neutropenia. A full blood count (FBC) should be done at six-monthly intervals, or more frequently, depending on the patient, to detect anaemia/neutropenia early. AZT can cause muscle pain or inflammation. AZT rarely causes hepatotoxicity, but may cause lactic acidosis.

Didanosine (ddI) may cause pancreatitis. Any patient presenting with abdominal pain should be investigated for pancreatitis. Peripheral neuropathy and lactic acidosis may also cause ddI.

Lopinavir/ritonavir is a combination drug. Both drugs are protease inhibitors. The major toxicities include lipid abnormalities and lipodystrophic change. Patients on this combination require six-monthly cholesterol and triglyceride analysis.

Potential side effects of the second-line regimen (Regimen 2)

The following are potential side effects of the second-line regimen (Regimen 2):

Bloating	Diarrhoea	Minor anaemia
Flatulence	Headache	Fatigue
Nausea	Vomiting	Weight loss

TREATMENT FAILURE

The definition of treatment failure depends on how the patient is monitored. A persistent increase in viral load after a period of suppression indicates virologic failure. A marked and persistent drop in CD4 count may also indicate failure.

A new opportunistic infection or a disease that changes the WHO staging of a patient who is already on antiretroviral therapy, would mean clinical failure. But, it is important to remember that new clinical events are common in the first three months after starting antiretroviral therapy and are not an indication for changing therapy. These clinical changes are often due to immune reconstitution syndrome, which is a syndrome that develops because improving immune function may unmask previously occult opportunistic infections, such as TB.

When viral loads and CD4 counts are not available, clinical monitoring alone is used to evaluate treatment failure or success.

If there is any one of virologic, CD4 count or clinical treatment failure, existing treatment should be stopped and three new drugs should be started.

SIDE EFFECTS OF ANTIRETROVIRAL THERAPY

The most common side effects of antiretroviral therapy include:

- skin rashes
- lactic acidosis
- hepatotoxicity
- hyperglycaemia, new onset diabetes mellitus, diabetic ketoacidosis and exacerbation of existing diabetes mellitus
- fat redistribution or a 'pseudo-Cushing's syndrome'
- hyperlipidaemia
- bone marrow suppression
- peripheral neuropathy
- nephrotoxicity
- diarrhoea
- ocular effects
- gastrointestinal intolerance
- headache
- insomnia.

Adverse effects can be due to short-term or long-term antiretroviral treatment. Short-term adverse reactions include nausea, diarrhoea and vomiting. These short-term side effects are significant as they can make the patient stop treatment and so cause poor adherence, which ultimately results in treatment failure.   Long-term adverse reactions include lipodystrophic syndrome, hyperlipidaemia associated with myocardial infarction and bone toxicity.

Adverse events are common; 41% of patients on the triple therapy regimen may experience them. Most (88%) of the adverse reactions are mild to moderate. The most common adverse reaction is elevated liver enzymes (AST/ALT more than three times the upper limit of normal). Another common adverse reaction is anaemia (Hb <9.5g/dl). Severe adverse reactions include bone marrow suppression, hepatotoxicity, and neuropsychiatric disorders. However, only 1.2% of patients on antiretrovirals experience serious adverse reactions. Serious adverse reactions may results in hospital admission, death or permanent disability (*Churchyard & Metcalf 2005*).

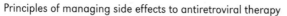

Principles of managing side effects to antiretroviral therapy

The following are principles of managing side effects to antiretroviral therapy:

- Establish whether the side effect is due to the antiretroviral drug or due to other medication.
- Consult an HIV specialist before changing or stopping antiretroviral therapy.
- If antiretroviral therapy needs to be stopped, all the drugs should be stopped at the same time.
- Never stop only one antiretroviral drug.
- Continue and closely observe antiretroviral therapy if the adverse reaction is mild. Stop antiretroviral therapy if the adverse reaction is severe.
- Adverse events should be recorded and reported to the National Adverse Drug Events Monitoring Centre.

Side effects and management of side effects

The management of the side effects has been adapted from the International Association of Physicians in AIDS Care (IAPAC) GRIP Guidelines. The IAPAC GRIP Guidelines are specially designed for clinicians and allied health professionals to use as reference material for the initiation and management of patients on antiretroviral therapy. The IAPAC GRIP guidelines are based on the Clinical Guidelines for Antiretroviral Therapy in Adults, March 2005.

Peripheral neuropathy

Consider discontinuing the drug causing the peripheral neuropathy (e.g. stavudine). The decision to discontinue a particular drug requires careful consideration. When in doubt refer the patient to an HIV specialist. If the decision is made to substitute, stavudine may be substituted with AZT. However, prior to starting AZT, test the patient's haemoglobin levels. Remember that the co-administration of stavudine with anti-TB treatment could precipitate peripheral neuropathy.

Pancreatitis

Should the patient develop pancreatitis, all the antiretroviral drugs should be discontinued. Ideally the patient should be referred to a specialist for further treatment.

Severe rash

Most rashes accompanying antiretroviral therapy are mild and usually resolve spontaneously even if the drug is continued. However, severe rashes include Stevens-Johnson syndrome, toxic epidermal necrolysis, abacavir hypersensitivity reaction rash and drug-related rash accompanied by eosinophilia and systemic symptoms.

The NNRTIs may be responsible for a severe rash. This rash usually occurs within the first two to four weeks of treatment. As nevirapine is frequently responsible for rashes, it is started only daily in both adults and children. If tolerated, the dose is increased to twice daily after two weeks. During this period it is important that the patient is told of the risks associated with any rash that develops and is closely monitored. Should the patient develop a severe rash on nevirapine, an HIV specialist should be consulted, who may recommend substituting the nevirapine. But nevirapine cannot be substituted with efavirenz as cross-sensitivity may occur.

If the rash is accompanied by fever, blisters, cutaneous bullae, mucosal lesions, systemic symptoms and/or elevated liver enzymes, it is recommended that all drugs be discontinued and the patient should be hospitalised and referred to a specialist.

Lactic acidosis

Lactic acidosis is a serious life-threatening complication of NRTIs, particularly didanosine and stavudine. Suspect lactic acidosis in a patient presenting with nausea, vomiting, abdominal pain, fatigue, a cough and/or shortness of breath. Lactic acidosis may also cause neurological symptoms similar to Guillain-Barré Syndrome.

A diagnosis of lactic acidosis is confirmed when the serum lactate is more than 5 mmol/l and the patient presents with a high anion gap metabolic acidosis. In certain instances, the liver enzymes may be elevated. Lactic acidosis may also occur due to immune reconstitution syndrome. Discontinue all drugs in patients presenting with lactic acidosis and refer to a specialist. Patients presenting with lactic acidosis may require ICU admission, and they require respiratory support and intravenous administration of fluids. Elevated liver enzymes and lactate levels take months to normalise.

Lipodystrophic changes

Lipodystrophy is the accumulation of fat on the abdomen (central obesity) on the face (moon face) and on the dorsocervical area (buffalo hump). This fat accumulation may be accompanied by lipoatrophy (loss of subcutaneous fat) on the extremities. Lipodystrophic changes may be reversible following discontinuation of antiretroviral therapy. Lipodystrophic change may occur due to treatment with lopinavir/ritonavir and stavudine.

Liver toxicity

All three drug classes, and particularly NNRTIs, may cause liver toxicity. Furthermore, the HIV infection itself may cause liver toxicity, and co-infection with hepatitis B and C, opportunistic infections, malignancies and drug interactions may also cause liver toxicity. For this reason liver enzymes should be monitored. If the ALT levels increase to five times greater than normal, all drugs should be discontinued and specialist referral sought. Adults are more likely to get liver toxicity than children.

Confusion, psychosis or depression

Efavirenz may cause confusion, psychosis or depression and this drug is avoided in individuals with a history of a psychiatric condition, but these reactions may occur in previously normal people. Should the patient develop severe depression, have suicidal ideation or psychosis they should be referred for specialist psychiatric management.

Severe anaemia

Severe anaemia may occur as a result of treatment with AZT. Severe anaemia may also be caused by HIV infection, AIDS-related conditions, such as disseminated *Mycobacterium avium*, cytomegalovirus, lymphoma or nutritional deficiencies. Severe anaemia is defined as a haemoglobin of less than 8 g/dl. Prior to starting AZT treatment the patient's haemoglobin levels should be measured. AZT should be discontinued if the patient is very pale or has a low haemoglobin (<8 g/dl). AZT may be substituted with stavudine in anaemic patients.

Neutropenia

Neutropenia is more common in children than in adults. Frequently, mild neutropenia will resolve spontaneously, unless it is accompanied by persistent fever and localised infection.

Hypersensitivity syndrome

Abacavir and nevirapine are the drugs that most often cause hypersensitivity syndrome. Hypersensitivity caused by abacavir typically presents as systemic illness accompanied by fever, rash, nausea, vomiting, diarrhoea, fatigue, myalgia and arthralgia. Respiratory symptoms, similar to those of a respiratory tract infection, may be present. About 70% of patients presenting with hypersensitivity syndrome will have a maculopapular or urticarial rash. Hypersensitivity syndrome occurs most often in the first six weeks of treatment. Hypersensitivity syndrome is fully reversible on discontinuation of the offending drug. However, the patient must never be rechallenged with the drug, as this may be fatal.

Hyperlipidaemia

The protease inhibitors are the main antiretrovirals implicated in causing hyperlipidaemia. However, both stavudine and efavirenz can also cause hyperlipidaemia. Hyperlipidaemia in adults could result in cardiovascular complications. Patients presenting with hyperlipidaemia should ideally be referred to a dietician and start a healthy eating plan, accompanied with exercise.

SAFETY MONITORING

Various blood tests are necessary for the duration of antiretroviral therapy to ensure the safety of the treatment:

- The CD4 count should be monitored six to 12 monthly.
- Liver enzymes (ALT) should be monitored as follows:
  - two weeks after commencing nevirapine
  - four weeks after commencing nevirapine
  - eight weeks after commencing nevirapine
  - every six months thereafter.
- A pregnancy test is necessary before starting efavirenz as this drug is teratogenic.
- Fasting glucose, triglycerides and cholesterol should be measured regularly.
- Monitor haemoglobin levels of patients on AZT prior to starting treatment and then six to 12 monthly.

DRUG INTERACTIONS

There are multiple opportunities for severe drug interactions between antiretroviral therapy and other drugs. The following drug interactions should be considered when managing a patient on antiretroviral therapy:

- Rifampicin (anti-TB drug) reduces the blood levels of nevirapine and these two drugs should not be used together.

- Efavirenz reduces the therapeutic blood levels of clarithromycin, but efavirenz can be given with azithromycin (both are macrolide antibiotics).

- Children with epilepsy should preferably be managed on sodium valproate as this drug is the safest of the antiepileptics when used with antiretrovirals.

- Drugs that are metabolised by cytochrome P450 have the potential for multiple drug interactions. These drugs include: ritonavir, lopinavir, efavirenz, and nevirapine.

DRUG RESISTANCE

HIV is highly adaptable and capable of changing its form. The ability of the HI virus to mutate is its key to survival. Through subtle changes in the genetic structure of the virus, it is able to evade attack by the immune system. Likewise the virus is also able to evade attack by antiretroviral drugs, thus making treatment of HIV and development of a vaccination difficult.

Viral resistance to any one antiviral drug has increased from 5.5% in 1998 to 14.5% in 2003. Most observed drug resistance is to nucleoside and non-nucleoside reverse transcriptase inhibitors (James & Nelson 2005). As a result, in the developed world, individual resistance testing is routine prior to the initiation of antiretroviral therapy. However, in South Africa, such testing is too expensive for general use.

IMMUNE RECONSTITUTION DISEASE

Immune reconstitution disease is the paradoxical clinical deterioration that occurs in a patient after they have started antiretroviral therapy. Immune reconstitution disease occurs due to the improving immune system interacting with organisms that have colonised the body during the early stages of HIV infection. It is important to differentiate immune reconstitution disease from treatment failure.

Immune reconstitution disease may be due to infection with *Mycobacterium tuberculosis, Mycobacterium avium complex, Mycobacterium leprae, Aspergillus fumigatus, Candida albicans, Pneumocystis jiroveci,* cytomegalovirus, human herpes virus, hepatitis B and hepatitis C.

Immune reconstitution syndrome usually occurs within the first six weeks following the start of highly active antiretroviral therapy. The clinical presentation of immune reconstitution syndrome will vary depending on the type of infecting organism and the organ affected.

Immune reconstitution syndrome is distressing for patients as they think that the antiretroviral therapy they have recently started is failing. This may result in poor adherence to treatment and must be explained carefully.

THE COST OF ANTIRETROVIRAL THERAPY

An evaluation of the cost of antiretroviral therapy includes the costs of provision of the healthcare service, the value of changes to healthcare utilisation and cost savings due to decreased labour turnover, decreased absenteeism and increased employee productivity (*Churchyard & Metcalf 2005*). The average total cost per patient on antiretrovirals per month in 2004 was R1 234. Drug and laboratory costs accounted for 65% of the costs. After two years of treatment, costs decreased to less than R1 000.

Studies have shown that patients on antiretroviral treatment generally experience a 60% reduction in illness-related absenteeism within the first 12 months of starting antiretroviral therapy. This reduced absenteeism results in a cost saving of R725 per employee per month of antiretroviral treatment. Furthermore, patients on antiretrovirals generally reduce the number of in-patient and out-patient visits. The reduction in patient visits results in a healthcare saving of R1 120 per employee on treatment for one month. Therefore, the cost of providing antiretroviral therapy is offset by the resultant reduction in healthcare utilisation (*Churchyard & Metcalf 2005*).

ADHERENCE TO ANTIRETROVIRAL THERAPY

The definition of adherence

What is adherence?

Adherence to antiretroviral therapy implies that the HIV and AIDS patient must take at least 95% of their doses of antiretroviral therapy; therefore they should not miss more than three doses in one month. If adherence is less than 80% that patient is at risk of experiencing failure of virological suppression and at increased risk of developing drug resistance.

Adherence to antiretroviral therapy is essential

Why is adherence to antiretroviral therapy essential?

Adherence to antiretroviral therapy is essential for the following reasons:

- It is necessary to ensure the long-term benefits of antiretroviral therapy.

- It is necessary to ensure that the antiretroviral drugs are effective.
- It is essential to prevent the development of drug resistance.

Requirements for adherence

The following strategies aid adherence to antiretroviral therapy:

- A comprehensive adherence plan.
- Implementation of multiple adherence strategies.
- Disclosure to a trusted individual.
- Multidisciplinary and multisectoral involvement.
- Community support, social support and support groups.
- People living with AIDS sharing adherence strategies.

Barriers to adherence

A new diagnosis of HIV and AIDS or disease progression can be a barrier to adherence. The development of an opportunistic infection could result in poor adherence as the patient may feel despondent, or the patient may feel that the antiretroviral therapy is failing. This may even result in depression. Should the individual require admission for the treatment of an opportunistic infection, they may not disclose that they are on antiretroviral therapy, resulting in discontinuation of antiretroviral therapy. In addition, the treatment of their opportunistic infection may result in drug interactions. Such drug interactions may necessitate a 'drug holiday' which is prescribed and monitored by an HIV specialist.

Death or trauma in the family may affect adherence. A death or trauma in the family may result in the individual on antiretroviral therapy having to travel away from their clinic and miss appointments. Death in the family may also raise financial concerns, which could affect access to health care.

Depression affects adherence. Depression results in reduced motivation and in apathy. The HIV-positive individual on antiretroviral therapy may lose the motivation to take their medication.

Trust is required for adherence. Trust affects adherence in many ways. Firstly, the HIV-positive individual on antiretroviral therapy should disclose their HIV status and the fact that they are on medication to a trusting partner. The trusting partner is an individual selected by the patient and may be a spouse, mother, father, child or any other relative or friend. This individual serves as their social support. In addition, the patient needs to trust the healthcare team in order to adhere to antiretroviral therapy. The patient needs to trust that the antiretroviral therapy will improve their quality of life. Finally, the HIV and AIDS-infected individual needs to trust the government and the healthcare system. Nurses who are not convinced that antiretroviral therapy is effective in improving quality of life for the HIV and AIDS-infected individual may consciously or unconsciously negatively influence their patients, resulting in lack of trust and poor adherence.

Trauma or intensive care admission reduces adherence. A patient who has sustained trauma and requires hospital admission is unable to inform healthcare professionals of their antiretroviral therapy, particularly if they are unconscious. As a result antiretroviral therapy will be unintentionally stopped. Antiretroviral therapy may intentionally be stopped should the patient become seriously ill and require intensive care admission as many drug interactions may occur. This intentional 'drug holiday' is prescribed and monitored by an HIV specialist doctor.

Immune reconstitution syndrome affects adherence. If immune reconstitution syndrome is not clearly explained to patients they may think that their antiretroviral therapy is failing and may not adhere to treatment.

'Pill fatigue' is the barrier to adherence that develops over time. Adherence may wane over time, even in highly adherent patients, so adherence should be monitored at every possible opportunity.

Irresponsible use of antiretroviral therapy is a barrier to adherence. It is the responsibility of the nurse to keep up-to-date with treatment strategies, thus ensuring the safe and responsible use of antiretroviral therapy.

Illiteracy and language problems are a barrier to adherence. Poor literacy and language problems impede understanding of the important of adherence to antiretroviral therapy and thus adherence.

Anxiety and other psychological problems reduce adherence. Anxiety about the antiretroviral therapy based on previous personal experience or experience of a family member or friend impedes adherence.

Strategies to ensure adherence

The nurse is an important point of contact for the patient, and thus performs the most important role in ensuring and maintaining adherence. The following are ways of promoting adherence:

Multiple contacts and ongoing education are essential in adherence to antiretroviral therapy. Adherence should be assessed at every possible opportunity and education on adherence should be provided. Within the current antiretroviral programme in South Africa the nurse has at least three appointment opportunities to either personally provide adherence counselling or to refer the patient to a counsellor for adherence counselling.

This occurs prior to the initiation of antiretroviral therapy. Following the initiation of antiretroviral therapy the nurse should ensure that the patient receives adherence counselling at each follow-up appointment. This ongoing adherence counselling is especially important once the patient has been on antiretroviral medication for a prolonged period of time due to the negative effects of 'pill fatigue'. In addition, should there be any change in the patient's physical, psychological and social circumstances, step-up adherence counselling should be considered.

Support and a non-judgemental attitude by the nurse are important for adherence. A nurse who is supportive and approaches the patient with a non-judgemental attitude is more likely to obtain an accurate assessment of the patient's barriers to adherence and to notice possible drug interactions. Patients may be taking other medication and not disclosing this information due to fear. If they feel supported and do not feel judged, they are more likely to disclose either poor adherence or the use of complementary and alternative medicine (CAM).

Reduce the pill burden. Treatment that requires a number of different pills to be taken at different times of the day is said to have a high pill burden and is more likely to result in reduced adherence. Combination treatments are being developed that reduce the pill burden and therefore result in improved adherence.

Treat side effects of antiretroviral therapy and opportunistic infections timeously. Side effects and opportunistic infections can negatively affect adherence. The patient should understand that they should report side effects and other infections timeously so that they can receive treatment. Patients should be discouraged from stopping treatment prior to consultation with an HIV specialist doctor.

Provide understandable and comprehensive information on HIV and AIDS and on antiretroviral therapy. It is critical that the nurse provides clear and comprehensible information to patients on all aspects of antiretroviral therapy and adherence. Information should be organised and structured to improve understanding and recall. Avoid complicated medical jargon. Repeat important statements or instructions. Provide the opportunity for the patient to repeat the instruction. Written instructions are useful. It is important that any myths and untruths are investigated and corrected.

Trust is important for adherence. Satisfaction with the nurse–patient interaction is an important contributing factor towards adherence. Patients are more likely to adhere if they feel that they can trust their nurse and if the nurse is caring and empathetic. Truth telling on the part of the nurse is critical to ensure patient trust. Patients should not carry the false belief that antiretroviral therapy will cure their HIV. Furthermore, facilitate a positive nurse-patient interaction through providing the patient with the opportunity to ventilate their fears and feelings about the treatment and ensure empathetic listening. Praise and encouragement reduce anxiety and improve belief in personal ability.

Reduce anxiety and improve the nurse-patient interaction. Anxiety experienced by the patient during the nurse-patient interaction reduces the patient's ability to retain information. This means that interaction should occur in a trusting, supportive and non-judgemental environment.

Avoid disruption caused by antiretroviral treatment. The more a treatment disrupts a patient's lifestyle the less likely they are to adhere to it. Structure treatment so that it results in minimal disruption to the patient's lifestyle. One factor that results in disruption to lifestyle is complexity of the treatment. Structure treatment in such a way that it is simple for the patient to follow and integrate into their normal activities of daily living.

Always obtain informed consent. Obtaining informed consent from the patient prior to commencing antiretroviral therapy is a vital aspect of adherence. While obtaining informed consent, assess the patient's understanding of antiretroviral therapy and the need for adherence.

Ensure the internal locus of control. Passive participation of patients in their antiretroviral regimen is not encouraged. Patients who feel that they are in control of their treatment are more likely to adhere. Insight into the disease, the disease process, the role of treatment and prognosis are all necessary to ensure insight, which is required for an internal locus of control.

Ongoing professional development is vital in the nursing profession. Healthcare professionals are required to keep up to date with the latest developments in antiretroviral therapy. They too require constant reminders on the importance of adherence.

Multisectoral collaboration is necessary to ensure adherence. The sectors that may be involved include non-governmental organisations, faith-based organisations, community-based organisations and employers who all have a vital role to perform in ensuring adherence. Inform patients about the importance of adherence and be sensitive to the interventions required to ensure adherence.

DOTS is the directly observed treatment strategy used in the Tuberculosis Control Programme. The methods of DOTS are useful in ensuring adherence to antiretroviral therapy. However, TB treatment is short term and antiretroviral therapy is for life.

Important information for adherence

Accurate and understandable instructions are an important tool for adherence. Give patients the following important information about their antiretroviral therapy:

- the name and purpose of the drugs, stressing the positive effects of the antiretroviral therapy
- the frequency and timing of drug administration according to normal daily routine
- a description of route of administration and special administration requirements
- the importance of not stopping therapy
- how and when to obtain the next supply
- any anticipated adverse reactions including: duration, self-management and when to seek medical attention for adverse reactions.

Reinforce the fact that the proposed duration of therapy is lifelong.

Special tests will be conducted to monitor side effects. The patient is advised not to stop treatment due to adverse reactions unless under the instruction of a doctor.

Adherence counselling

Adherence counselling should ideally be conducted in the following manner:

- Spend time explaining all three drugs included in the antiretroviral therapy.
- Monitor adherence to other medication (e.g. prophylactic co-trimoxazole) for one month prior to administering antiretroviral therapy.
- Negotiate a treatment plan with the patient that is understandable and practical.
- Encourage the patient to disclose their HIV status to a person whom they can trust and who will act as a support person.
- Inform the patient of potential side effects and the management of the side effects.
- Establish prior to initiating antiretroviral therapy whether this is in fact the patient's wish and whether the patient is ready for it.
- Provide adherence tools, such as tick charts, reminders or marked pill boxes.
- Encourage the use of alarms as reminders.

- Avoid drug interactions by ensuring a thorough knowledge of the patient's regimen and other medication the patient may be taking.
- Anticipate, monitor and treat side effects.
- Include the patient in adherence discussion groups and support groups.

Step-up adherence

Step-up adherence strategies are employed if poor adherence or a barrier to adherence is identified. Consider the following steps when implementing step-up adherence.

- Identify and investigate the barrier.
- Increase the frequency of clinic visits until adherence is ensured.
- Enlist the support of a person identified by the patient. This person may even need to be brought into the clinic for adherence counselling. (This can only be done with the consent of the patient).
- Review the patient's knowledge, correct misconceptions and re-educate.

INFECTION CONTROL ISSUES

Ansie Minnaar

Throughout the AIDS epidemic, nosocomial infections in patients with HIV diseases have presented a constant problem.

(Laing 1999)

INTRODUCTION

HIV-positive patients are more likely to suffer from nosocomial infections than HIV-negative patients. HIV-positive patients are at an increased risk of acquiring nosocomial infections in hospitals and other healthcare institutions. Because of the risk that nosocomial infections pose to HIV-positive patients, you need to understand specific risk factors and the control measures that need to be implemented in hospitals and other healthcare facilities. The exact

HIV seroprevalence rates among patients in South African hospitals are not known. However, there are a few factors that need to be considered when we are managing nosocomial infections in a hospital. The numbers of HIV and AIDS patients are increasing in our hospitals. Potential contamination of water supplies adds to the problem of infection control. HIV-positive patients in hospital are at risk of a wider range of opportunistic infections and also of nosocomial infections, because they are immunocompromised. Furthermore, contamination of the hospital environment by organisms such as *Clostridium difficile* and *Cryptosporidium parvum* and *Mycobacterium avium complex* is particularly dangerous for patients with HIV (*Duse 1999*).

RESPIRATORY INFECTIONS

Nosocomial tuberculosis (TB) was reported before the HIV epidemic started, but nosocomial TB in HIV-positive patients increases the risk of active TB developing, with an accelerated course of the disease (*Laing 1999*). The spread of multidrug-resistant TB between HIV-positive patients is a huge concern, as is its possible spread to healthcare workers. The delay in recognition of multidrug-resistant TB, and therefore the delayed initiation of effective drug therapy, and poor infection control measures to prevent the spread of the infection, are major factors in the spread of nosocomial multidrug-resistant TB. Studies have shown that the best way to prevent the spread of TB between patients and between patients and healthcare workers is the introduction of strict isolation facilities in negative pressure rooms until that patient produces at least three negative sputum samples. Nebulised therapy and physiotherapy should be conducted in adapted respiratory isolation rooms, which allow sufficient air exchange to remove possible airborne particles between patients and patients, and patients and staff.

Gram-negative nosocomial pneumonias in HIV-positive patients are known to have been caused by organisms such as *Klebsiella*, *Enterobacter* and *Pseudomonas*. *Staphylococcus aureus*, *Streptococcus pneumoniae* and *Haemophilus influenzae* and *Streptococcus viridans* have also been identified as pathogens in patients with HIV infection (*Laing 1999*).

Pseudomonas infections in HIV-positive patients are most common in the lungs and are probably caused by person-to-person contact.

Nosocomial infections may also spread from AIDS patients to other immunocompromised patients, such as those with cancer. *Pneumocystis jiroveci* pneumonia has been reported among cancer patients since the start of the HIV pandemic.

Other nosocomial infections in patients with HIV infection

Staphylococcus areus infections are probably the most common causative agent of nosocomial infections in HIV-positive patients. This is probably the result of a combination of the skin entrance of Staphylococcus together with the frequent use of central vascular catheters (CVCs).

Bacteraemia in HIV-positive patients is known to be a significant problem. Studies have shown that CVCs and urinary catheters are used significantly more often in HIV-positive patients. Bloodstream infection caused most of the nosocomial infections, followed by urinary tract infections, vascular infections and pneumonia. There is also some evidence to suggest that HIV patients may be a reservoir of methacillin-resistant *Staphylococcus areus* (MRSA) in hospitals.

Other important nosocomial infections are *Klebsiella pneumoniae* and *Pseudomonas aeruginosa*.

Furthermore, the breakdown in integrity of the skin as a consequence of Kaposi's sarcoma and dermatoses leads to increased susceptibility to staphylococcal and gram-negative infections. Invasive procedures and indwelling devices may be associated with bacteraemia and fungaemia. Neoplasms may be associated with a variety of organisms such as clostridia, enterococci, *S. bovis* and gram-negative infections (*Padoveze et al. 2002*).

PREVENTION STRATEGIES

Risk factors for bacterial colonisation and infection include immuno-suppression, prior treatment with an antibiotic, increased hospitalisation with longer lengths of stay and greater exposure to invasive devices. These factors all contribute to higher infection rates in hospitals and healthcare facilities.

Hand washing and hand disinfection should be compulsory in any hospital or healthcare facility. Plastic aprons should be used in case of secretions and a mask in case of splashes. Laundry, waste and cleaning should be done according to standard infection control precautionary measures, appropriate to the patient's condition. Patients with AIDS and additional infections should be nursed in a single room with universal precautions against contamination by blood and secretions (*Duse 1999*).

Potential occupational exposure

The following should be regarded as occupational risks:

- needle stick or sharp injuries (used needles or sharps)
- splashes of infectious body fluids onto mucous membranes

- accidental penetrative injuries, for example, patient bite wounds
- contamination by blood.

Potentially exposed employees

Employees working in a healthcare facility are exposed to certain risky tasks and procedures and need to take universal precautions in the following circumstances:

- during blood collection and the use of sharp instruments, such as needles and certain catheters
- during the insertion of intravenous catheters
- during minor and major surgery
- when handling soiled linen
- when handling corpses and being involved in post mortem examinations (*Ziady et al. 1997*).

Health professionals should have information about prevention programmes and adopt the following measures to prevent percutaneous injuries during all patient contacts:

- wash hands after any direct contact with a patient
- wear personal protective equipment such as gloves, a protective gown and a mask
- cover any cuts and abrasions
- have hepatitis B immunization
- avoid recapping needles following invasive procedures
- dispose of sharps according to universal infection control measures
- avoid fatigue and working long hours
- treat all patients as HIV positive and use universal infection control measures
- avoid using fingers to receive the needle while suturing and rather use forceps and a needle holder
- concentrate and pay attention
- receive ongoing education and reinforcement of universal precautions and prevention strategies in all healthcare settings (*Bodkin & Bruce 2003*).

Theatre staff should take particular care and should not receive suture needles in their hands.

Recommendations for post-exposure prophylaxis (PEP)

Post-exposure prophylaxis is recommended for high-risk exposure. See Tables 13.1 and 13.2 for PEP regimens for different risk exposures. Staff in healthcare facilities must be trained in how to handle exposure to high-risk patients.

Furthermore, supportive counselling must be available to staff in case of exposure to HIV-infected patients. An ELISA test should be done on the exposed healthcare worker within 24 hours of exposure, and again after six weeks, twelve weeks and after six months, if the initial test is negative. All injuries should be reported to the direct supervisor within one hour and within 24 hours to the nursing service manager of the health services, to the occupational health centre within one to two hours, and within seven days to the Compensation Commissioner and to the Provincial Head of Occupational health within a month.

Type of occupational exposure, risk of exposure, HIV status of the source and recommendations for PEP

Table 5.1		Percutaneous injury	Risk of exposure	Recommendations for PEP
	1	Superficial injury	Some risk	Consider basic regimen
	2	Skin puncture, visible blood on the needle	High risk	Recommend basic regimen
	3	Needle used in vein or artery or injection into body	Highest risk	Recommend basic regimen and expanded regimen
	4	Deep intra-muscular injury or injection into the body	Highest risk	Recommend basic regimen and expanded regimen
		Skin contact	**Risk of exposure**	**Recommendations for PEP**
	5	Unbroken healthy skin	Low risk/no risk	Not recommended
	6	Compromised skin, small volume and brief contact	Low risk	Consider basic regimen
	7	Compromised skin, large volume and prolonged contact	Increased risk	Consider basic regimen

	HIV status of source	Risk of exposure	Recommendations for PEP
8	Negative	Very low	Not recommended
9	HIV positive, clinical AIDS and/or low CD4 count	Low for small volumes or short duration on intact skin	Consider basic regimen
10	HIV positive, clinical AIDS and/or low CD4 count	High risk for percutaneous injuries	Recommend basic regime and expanded regimen
11	Unknown		Consider PEP on a case by case basis

Source: Department of Health, Gauteng Provincial Government: Guidelines for prophylaxis for accidental exposure to blood borne pathogens. In-house publication

Recommended PEP drug regimes

Drug	Dose	Frequency	Duration
Zidovudine (AZT)	200 mg	8 hourly	4 weeks
Lamivudine (3TC)	150 mg	12 hourly	4 weeks
For very high-risk exposures – add indinavir	800 mg	8 hourly	4 weeks

Table 5.2

Source: Department of Health, Gauteng Provincial Government: Guidelines for prophylaxis for accidental exposure to blood borne pathogens. In-house publication

CONCLUSION

The introduction of antiretroviral treatment, and so prolonged survival of HIV and AIDS patients, will force improved infection control measures and surveillance of nosocomial infections in the future in all healthcare facilities in South Africa. It also seems probable that health workers will increasingly be faced with the challenge of prevention and diagnosis of nosocomial infections as the HIV and AIDS epidemic progresses.

CHAPTER 6

LIVING POSITIVELY WITH HIV AND AIDS, PATIENT MANAGEMENT AND COMMUNICATION

Ansie Minnaar

> Some people walk in the rain.
>
> Others just get wet.
>
> *(Roger Miller in Kelly-Heidenthal 2003)*

INTRODUCTION

All of us live with AIDS. Some of us have HIV, and others full-blown AIDS, others are HIV negative. However, all of us, as members of a society and global village, are interconnected with the realities of HIV and AIDS. People living with AIDS (PLWAs) is a well-known concept in nursing. Because members of every community are infected with HIV, changes need to be made in healthcare delivery as well as health and other education, to cope with prevention strategies and new medication. Social services and the law are changing in ways that are necessary to fight the HIV and AIDS epidemic in South Africa. The HIV and AIDS pandemic has forced people to confront the realities of both homosexual and heterosexual sex. The purpose of this chapter, however, is to address the human dimensions of HIV and AIDS.

The experiences and expectations of people living with HIV and AIDS

People living with HIV and AIDS have significant psychological, social, and physical challenges when dealing with their disease. When a person first learns that they are HIV positive, their self-concept is under pressure. Our self-concept is a social construct and is developed through our interactions with other people. Many people go into denial when they learn that they are HIV positive. However, most will confide in their closest family or friends. This step is never easy and may lead to thoughts such as: 'Will they think we are diseased, and never see us again?' 'Will they still love us?' 'Will they still have sexual relationships with us if we use condoms?' These questions raise issues of role expectations. The problem for the HIV-positive individual is that he or she does not know in advance how friends and family will react to and accommodate the news of their status (*Fan et al. 2000*).

Accepting the reality of infection

Each HIV-positive person eventually begins to accept the reality of HIV infection. Each individual's self-concept adjusts and roles change. The process of role adjustment involves risks, such as dealing with issues of tension in relationships, unrealistic hopes and dreams and the reality of unattainable goals. The process of adjustment is usually not easy and for some it is never completed or resolved. Although people with other life-threatening diseases also have a difficult path of acceptance, those with HIV and AIDS frequently have other challenges due to the stigma associated with HIV infection (*Fan et al. 2000*).

PEOPLE'S PRECONCEIVED ATTITUDES ABOUT OTHERS

Two concepts are important when we try to understand what it is like for people living with HIV and AIDS – namely, prejudice and discrimination (*Fan et al. 2000*). Prejudice is a biased attitude toward a group of people and it arises from people associating with particular groups of people or individuals. Prejudice could be positive or negative. Positive prejudice usually refers to thinking that people are good. However, there is often negative prejudice against people living with HIV. Stereotypes also relate to prejudice, where stereotyping is the cognitive basis for prejudice. Because stereotyping is group based, the stereotypes are usually innacurate. Because HIV and AIDS first appeared in homosexual men, prejudice against homosexuals caused a negative reaction to the disease among many people. People who were infected with HIV were blamed for contracting their illness through what was perceived as unacceptable behaviour. However, over time, HIV was diagnosed in positively stereotyped groups, such as people who contracted it through a blood transfusion. This led to confused attitudes to the infection, because these people were 'innocent victims' of circumstance. However, there is still strong general prejudice against those with HIV and AIDS. This prejudice exerts a strong influence on society's attitude to people infected with HIV and suffering from AIDS, and frequently results in discrimination. Prejudice relates to attitude and discrimination relates to actions. However, in South Africa, there is legislation against discrimination against those living with HIV, and HIV status cannot be used as grounds for dismissal from work or as a reason for not employing someone.

Emotional support and stress prevention

Patients with HIV and AIDS need emotional support to cope with the particular challenges they face. A person living with HIV may find that he or she is an outcast within the community, the workplace and in their family. With the correct lifestyle and access to antiretrovirals the patient can live a healthy life for many years and nurses need to acknowledge their role in helping the patient to cope and to live positively.

The stigma surrounding HIV and AIDS and the fear of rejection could affect the mental state of the patient, requiring counselling and continued support. Patients affected by HIV and AIDS may be concerned about losing their jobs because of their HIV status, particularly if they are ill and frequently absent from work. They also have to worry about their families and financial responsibilities and particularly about their children. The patient will also have concerns about disclosure, because of the stigma surrounding the infection. They may need counselling on how to cope with this and with any rejection they may experience.

If antiretroviral drugs are not available, the patient will have concerns about dying and need information about community support and home-based care.

Maintaining a healthy body

A healthy body and a strong immune system are priorities for people living with HIV. Sleep and rest are important, as is exercise and good nutrition. It is a good idea to try to avoid contact with people with other infections and those living with HIV should have an influenza vaccination every winter.

Good basic hygiene at home is very important, as is avoiding excess alcohol and smoking, as these can further weaken the immune system. All infections should be treated as soon as possible and patients should consult with their clinics or doctor regularly.

Patients living with HIV should practise safe sex to reduce the risk of re-infection with a different strain of HIV. A patient infected with multiple strains of HIV has a higher chance of developing AIDS. Multiple infections can result in an increased viral load and a decreased CD4 count.

A healthy diet will strengthen the immune system. Patients should wash their hands before touching food. Raw fruit and vegetables should be rinsed thoroughly with water containing a teaspoon of lemon juice and salt to ensure that all micro-organisms are killed or removed from the food. Foods that can cause food poisoning, such as fish, meat, poultry and eggs should be thoroughly cooked at a high temperature and should never be eaten raw. All utensils must be washed with hot water and soap after a meal. Drinking water should always be from a safe source, otherwise water should be boiled before use.

Lastly, the HIV-positive patient should eat food high in protein, such as beans, meat, eggs and fish. Include plenty of fresh fruit and vegetables and nuts, including peanut butter, to help boost the immune system.

In patients who are suffering from AIDS-related illness and fatigue, high-energy foods such as rice, potatoes and milk will be helpful. More frequent meals could be offered when the patient is suffering from anorexia and other food absorption defects. Fermented foods such as yogurt and maas will assist with fighting Candida infections and with the general digestion of food. Dehydration should be avoided and if the patient is not eating well, he or she should be encouraged to drink water or fruit juices.

An example of a nursing care plan for HIV and AIDS patients with gastrointestinal disorders

Table 6.1

	Nursing diagnosis	Plan/Goal	Nursing interventions
1	Fluid volume deficit related to nausea, vomiting, diarrhoea or inadequate oral intake	Normal skin turgor and decreased frequency and amount of stools	• Hard sweets or chewing gum can stimulate saliva production if mouth is dry • Encourage patient to drink liquids between meals

	Nursing diagnosis	Plan/Goal	Nursing interventions
			• Monitor and record intake and output of patient • Monitor patient for evidence of electrolyte imbalance such as hypocalaemia, hypochloraemia, confusion and muscle weakness
2	Nutrition providing less than body requirements because of anorexia, dysphasia, mal-absorption or side effects of medication	The patient will eat 75% of prescribed diet and maintain current weight	• Provide the prescribed diet (low-residue, high-caloric and high-protein) in small meals • Offer nutritional supplementation between meals • Administer supplemental vitamins and minerals • Provide oral hygiene before and after meals • Administer anti-emetics prn • Weigh the patient daily • Advise the patient to keep a food record and to log signs and symptoms of diarrhoea, vomiting and anorexia
3	Impaired skin integrity, related to diarrhoea and malnutrition	The patient will maintain skin integrity	• Monitor stools of patient for blood, fat and undigested food

Nursing diagnosis	Plan/Goal	Nursing interventions
		• Monitor stool cultures for new infections • Protect peri-rectal area by keeping it clean and using a barrier cream • Avoid prolonged pressure on bony prominences • Provide a pressure relief mattress • Avoid wrinkles in the bedding

Source: White 2001

Nutritional support

Nutritional support is important in all stages of HIV and AIDS infection and should begin when the patient is first diagnosed. There is a direct relationship between nutritional status and outcome in HIV disease. A baseline nutritional assessment should be done at diagnosis and every six months thereafter. The assessment includes a diet history, the body weight, a visual appraisal of general health, and laboratory tests for fasting blood sugar and lipid profiles. Education about nutrition is a key element of HIV and AIDS care. However, in South Africa it is often more important to find out if the patient has regular access to food and the amount of money he or she has available to buy food. It is also important to get a full medical history and a medication profile if possible.

Good nutrition strengthens the immune system, prevents muscle loss and slows the progress of the disease. Nutritional status should be evaluated frequently and the patient should be encouraged to maintain their weight and eat a diet high in calories and protein. Nutritional supplements and eating between meals may also help patients to maintain their body weight and preserve lean muscle mass. This is a huge problem in South Africa, where most people affected by HIV and AIDS are among the poorest in the world (*HIV/AIDS Update 2004*). See Chapter 7 for more information on nutrition for HIV and AIDS patients.

Food and water safety

Food and water-borne infections are much more commonly found in those living with HIV and AIDS and are more dangerous. These patients must take precautions to protect themselves from infections, such as salmonella, listeria and cryptosporidium. Foods that are associated with food-borne illness include: unpasteurised milk, raw or undercooked poultry, meat and eggs, foods made with raw eggs (mayonnaise, hollandaise sauce, Caesar salad dressing, and cake dough), unpasteurised cheeses, and improperly packaged or canned foods. Again clean water is still a problem in South Africa for many of those living with HIV. Patients should be educated on basic hygiene and the importance of hand washing in their daily lives.

CONCLUSION

In Africa, all of us live with HIV. In South Africa, one of the greatest challenges for people living with HIV and AIDS is obtaining access to antiretrovirals. The majority of people affected by HIV in southern Africa live in extreme poverty, which brings its own challenges. Added to this, prevention efforts across the region seem to be failing and there are thousands of new HIV infections every day.

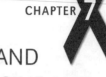

CHAPTER 7

COMPLEMENTARY AND ALTERNATIVE MEDICINE AND HIV AND AIDS MANAGEMENT

Candice Bodkin

KEY CONCEPTS

- complementary and alternative medicine
- traditional medicine
- herbal medicine
- nutritional considerations
- therapeutic touch
- vitamins
- minerals
- supplementation
- ethics

> The alternative management of HIV/AIDS infected individuals involves promoting psychological and physiological well-being as well as fostering socio-cultural relationships and supporting the fulfillment of spiritual aspirations
>
> *(Kinghorn and Gamlin 2001)*

INTRODUCTION

The HIV/AIDS/STI Strategic Plan for South Africa, 2000–2005 (*DOH 2000*), highlights three goals that relate to the integration of complementary and alternative medicine (CAM) and allopathic healthcare for the management of HIV and AIDS. Firstly, to improve the care and treatment of HIV-positive persons and persons living with AIDS in order to promote a better quality of life and limit the need for hospital care. Secondly, to collaborate with CAM practitioners in order to improve health-seeking behaviour. Finally, conduct research on the effectiveness of CAM. The importance of CAM and the need for collaboration between allopathic and CAM for the management of HIV and AIDS has been identified within the HIV/AIDS/STI Strategic Plan for South Africa, 2000–2005. It is for this reason that the integrated management of HIV and AIDS should be considered in South Africa.

In order to fully understand the process of integrating CAM and allopathic healthcare for the management of HIV and AIDS-infected individuals the following require clarification: the definitions of complementary and alternative medicine; the management of HIV and AIDS in the South African context; reasons for South African patients selecting CAM; the advantages and disadvantages of integrating CAM and allopathic healthcare in the South African context and guidelines for the safe and effective integration of alternative and allopathic healthcare for the management of HIV and AIDS-infected individuals. A detailed description of specific CAM therapies useful in the management of HIV and AIDS is included in this chapter.

DEFINITION OF ALTERNATIVE AND COMPLEMENTARY MEDICINE

HIV and AIDS is a complex disease that requires complex and holistic healthcare. One of the most significant benefits of integrating CAM and allopathic healthcare for the management of HIV and AIDS is the ability to provide holistic healthcare for HIV and AIDS-infected individuals in South Africa (*Knippels & Weiss 2000, de Visser et al. 2000*). The Canadian Holistic Medical Association defines holistic healthcare as, 'a system of healthcare which fosters a cooperative relationship among all those involved, leading towards optimal attainment of physical, psychological, social and spiritual well-being'. The provision of holistic healthcare is integral to the philosophy of alternative healthcare.

Complementary and alternative healthcare is defined as 'the scientific and non-scientific interventions that diverge from allopathic or western medicine for the treatment of HIV and AIDS. It is those practices explicitly used for the purpose of medical intervention, health promotion and disease prevention which are not routinely taught at health science faculties nor routinely underwritten by third party payers within the healthcare system'. CAM involves the non-invasive and non-pharmaceutical management of HIV and AIDS (*Kinghorn & Gamlin 2001*).

The alternative management of HIV and AIDS-infected individuals involves promoting psychological and physiological well-being, fostering socio-cultural relationships and supporting the fulfillment of spiritual aspirations (*Kinghorn & Gamlin 2001*).

Alternative healthcare in South Africa is provided in the form of traditional medicine. It is estimated that as many as 80% of the South African population seek traditional medicine (*Morris 2001*). Conversely allopathic healthcare, otherwise known as western medicine or modern medicine, involves invasive and pharmacological management of HIV and AIDS. Allopathic healthcare in the form of antiretroviral therapy is currently the management of choice for HIV and AIDS in South Africa.

HIV AND AIDS MANAGEMENT AND CAM IN SOUTH AFRICA

The National Health Plan for South Africa (1994) identified HIV and AIDS as a healthcare priority, and in addition identified the importance of the role that traditional and alternative healthcare play in the provision of healthcare to South Africans. Thus, the integration of alternative and allopathic healthcare for the management of HIV and AIDS is not a new concept. In fact, many organisations have developed the policies and resources required for the integration of alternative and allopathic healthcare. Such organisations include UNAIDS, the Commonwealth Working Group on Traditional and Complementary Health Systems and the Global Initiative for Traditional Systems of Health (*Morris 2001*).

The South African National HIV and AIDS programme, which followed the National Health Plan for South Africa in 1994, allowed for the establishment of a committee of traditional healers. The purpose of this committee was to look at the registration of all qualifying traditional healers, the promotion of training of traditional healers, professionalism and the creation of a traditional medicine data base. One other important function would be the coordination of collaboration between traditional healers and the allopathic healthcare system. Despite these initiatives alternative healthcare has received little obvious attention in South Africa (*Morris 2001*).

January 2000 saw the launch and implementation of the HIV/AIDS/STI Strategic Plan for South Africa, 2000–2005 (*DOH 2000*). This strategic plan advocates the comprehensive management of HIV and AIDS and includes HIV and AIDS treatment by means of antiretroviral therapy and the use of traditional medicine. The allopathic management of HIV and AIDS is based on a biomedical framework and involves combination therapy with antiretroviral therapy (*Wilson et al. 2002*).

WHY DO HIV AND AIDS-INFECTED INDIVIDUALS SELECT CAM?

HIV and AIDS-infected individuals select CAM for the following reasons:

- HIV and AIDS patients may become desperate. This is a result of the nature of the disease. Patients may seek assistance in any form to

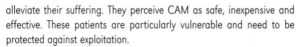

alleviate their suffering. They perceive CAM as safe, inexpensive and effective. These patients are particularly vulnerable and need to be protected against exploitation.

- A personal choice of healthcare offers the patient a sense of empowerment. The patient feels that by choosing their therapy they have more control over their illness. These patients are better educated and informed. These patients may also cope better with their illness because they may be less anxious and more able to make decisions about their healthcare.

- HIV and AIDS patients may distrust the medical establishment. This is particularly relevant to the South African situation because of the disputes between government and drug companies regarding the implementation of antiretroviral therapy. Research on HIV and AIDS prevention is slow and complicated. Patients may feel that it will be too late for them, so they take their healthcare into their own hands.

- Patients have easy access to complementary therapies. Most CAM products in South Africa are available within health stores or pharmacies without a prescription. These CAM medicines are cheap in comparison to antiretroviral therapies. Within the South African context CAM may be culturally acceptable, as many of the therapies used are traditional herbs and may be issued by traditional practitioners.

- Conventional antiretroviral therapies are viewed as expensive and toxic. Many patients abort antiretroviral therapy because of cost and side effects. Patients develop rapid resistance to antiretroviral therapy if adherence is poor. Antiretroviral therapy is indicated in South Africa, once the patient has reached a CD4 count of 200 cells/µl or less. HIV patients may use CAM if their CD4 count is greater than 200 cells/µl.

- Patients view CAM as non-toxic. However, not all CAM therapies are without side effects. Patients choosing CAM should be under the supervision of a registered practitioner, particularly if they are also on antiretrovirals or are in the advanced stages of the disease. CAM is particularly useful in the management of the following conditions in HIV and AIDS: persistent fatigue, skin rashes, persistent diarrhoea, persistent fever, headache, fungal infections, weight loss, soreness and burning of feet and legs, and depression (*Standish et al. 2001*).

ADVANTAGES OF THE USE OF CAM FOR THE MANAGEMENT OF HIV AND AIDS

The Department of Health (2000) recommends collaboration between CAM and allopathic healthcare in order to offer comprehensive HIV and AIDS management to South Africans. The integration of alternative and allopathic healthcare for the management of HIV and AIDS has many advantages in South Africa. CAM offers the ability to provide holistic and safe healthcare to HIV and AIDS-infected children. CAM may enhance immune function and can be used to manage the side effects of antiretroviral therapy. CAM can be used to complement antiretroviral therapy or can be used where antiretroviral therapy is not indicated. CAM can offer benefits to HIV-infected pregnant women in addition to the prevention of mother-to-child transmission (PMTC) of HIV. Finally, CAM provides an alternative when antiretroviral therapy is unavailable. Each advantage requires elaboration.

Complementary and alternative HIV and AIDS management for children

Children could benefit from CAM. In some children HIV infection progresses rapidly and these children need early treatment. Knowledge of how to treat children with HIV is often limited and there are fewer treatment options available. There is a real need both for the development of methods for the management of HIV and AIDS in children and for better education about the treatments that are currently available for children. Currently CAM may be used for the treatment of local and minor infections in HIV and AIDS-affected children (*Henderson 2001, Madsen et al. 2003*).

Complementary and alternative medicine and antiretroviral therapy

The HI virus is highly adaptable and its ability to mutate is the key to its survival. Mutation makes it possible for the virus to evade attack by the immune system and by antiretroviral therapy, thus making treatment of HIV and AIDS and formulation of a vaccination difficult (*Marcolin 2001*). Users of CAM maintain the belief that the therapies have an immune-stimulating function. In addition studies conducted on HIV and AIDS-infected CAM users maintain that while CAM does not provide a cure, it can improve quality of life (*Griffis et al. 2001, Hsiao et al. 2003*). Antiretroviral therapies reduce viral load initially but do not offer a cure for HIV and AIDS infection and studies show a viral rebound within 12 weeks of discontinuing antiretroviral treatment (*Bartlett & Gallant 2000*). This is especially true for HIV and AIDS patients who were taking antiretroviral therapy but have decided to discontinue. CAM can play an important role in improving the quality of life for these patients.

CAM can also be used where antiretroviral therapy is not indicated or the HIV and AIDS-infected individual chooses not to take conventional therapy. Antiretroviral therapy is offered to patients who have a CD4 count below 200 cells/μl or who are presenting with AIDS-related symptoms (*Bartlett & Gallant 2000*). CAM could be useful for HIV-infected individuals who have a CD4 count greater than 500 cells/μl. Some HIV and AIDS-infected individuals for whom antiretroviral therapy is indicted chose not to take the treatment or do not adhere to treatment. In order for antiretroviral therapy to be effective it should be taken every day for many years. Such therapy can result in lipodystrophy, hyperlipidaemia, metabolic disturbances, and reduced bone mineral density (*Bartlett & Gallant 2000*). These side effects sometimes result in poor adherence and a reluctance to commence antiretroviral therapy, resulting in increased drug resistance.

Complementary and alternative medicine and HIV-positive pregnant women

A single dose (200 mg) of nevirapine is provided to pregnant women at the onset of labour in public sector hospitals in South Africa as part of the PMTCT of HIV programme. This treatment reduces HIV transmission from mother to child. But nevirapine is not always available (*Morris 2001*). In addition, the single dose of nevirapine only benefits the child, because while it prevents the transmission of HIV from mother to child it does not benefit the health of the mother. There is a need for further research into the use of CAM that can safely be used during pregnancy, which could benefit the mother. These benefits include stimulating the immune system of the HIV-infected pregnant woman, and thus reducing poor maternal health outcomes, repeated minor HIV-related infections and complications during pregnancy.

Complementary and alternative medicine in the South African healthcare system

The process of distributing treatment to HIV-infected individuals has been slow, resulting in reduced trust in the medical fraternity (*Morris 2001, Sidley 2003*). HIV-infected individuals feel that time is running out. They feel that is it time for them to take responsibility for their health. CAM can provide the opportunity for a person to take responsibility for their own health (*Kinghorn & Gamlin 2001*).

THE DISADVANTAGES OF CAM FOR THE MANAGEMENT OF HIV AND AIDS

The disadvantages of the use of CAM for HIV and AIDS management in South Africa include concerns about poor adherence to antiretroviral therapy, concerns about patient safety and concerns about effectiveness and availability of CAM for the management of HIV and AIDS.

Patient safety and CAM

A thoughtful and well-trained practitioner should be the only person administering CAM to HIV and AIDS patients. A possible danger is that those using CAM may stop appropriate medical treatment, such as antiretroviral therapy, or prophylaxis for the prevention of opportunistic infection. In addition, if antiretroviral therapy or prophylaxis for opportunistic infection is substituted by CAM, there are concerns around the safety of the alternative therapies.

Efficacy of complementary and alternative therapies for the management of HIV and AIDS

The inclusion of CAM in the management of HIV and AIDS requires that, in certain circumstances, CAM is used in conjunction with antiretroviral therapy. Drug interactions can occur between homeopathy, herbal remedies and antiretroviral therapy, so CAM/allopathic combinations need to be selected with caution. Drug interactions between CAM and antiretroviral therapy may result in reduced efficacy of either the antiretroviral therapy or the CAM.

In addition to concerns about the safety of CAM, there is little evidence on the effectiveness of CAM, as there are few clinical trials.

The availability of complementary and alternative medicine for the management of HIV and AIDS in South Africa

There are questions and concerns surrounding the availability of CAM for the management of HIV and AIDS in South Africa. CAM is not included on the essential drugs list and thus cannot be supplied at a reduced cost, or to HIV and AIDS-infected individuals receiving care at public sector clinics or hospitals.

Availability is also affected by the fact that CAM has been marginalised, poorly regulated and undersubsidised. However, CAM remains widely used for the management of HIV and AIDS. This is because some HIV and AIDS-infected individuals view alternative health care as effective, safe, relatively cheap and improving quality of life (*Standish et al. 2001*).

CAM FOR THE MANAGEMENT OF HIV AND AIDS

The following are complementary and alternative therapies that may be useful in the management of HIV and AIDS:

- good nutrition
- vitamins, minerals and other supplements
- herbal medicine
- traditional medicine
- psychological and spiritual work
- Chinese medicine
- therapeutic activities.

Nutrition

There is plenty of research into the importance of nutrition in HIV and AIDS management. Many studies have shown the detrimental effects of weight loss on HIV and AIDS patients. Weight loss can result in increased morbidity and mortality.

The pathophysiology of weight loss in HIV and AIDS is complex. The theory is that certain cytokines cause inadequate utilisation of energy sources and prevent cells from absorbing nutrients. This is compounded by an increased metabolic rate, due to pyrexia and infection. Thus, the body requires more nutrients but has difficulty absorbing them. Inadequate nutrient intake and poor appetite exacerbate these problems. This results in malnutrition.

HIV and AIDS patients need early and aggressive nutritional programmes. It is important to intervene early with education and nutritional counselling. Establish baseline weight and nutritional status at the first visit and monitor weight fluctuations at subsequent visits.

An involuntary weight loss of more than 10% of body weight is AIDS-defining and weight loss is one of the more obvious symptoms of HIV and AIDS. Once the individual starts to lose weight they consider seeking medical attention, even if they have not already been diagnosed with HIV. Good nutrition in HIV and AIDS requires education.

This involuntary weight loss could be due to anorexia, nausea, vomiting, dyspnoea, fatigue, neurological disease and infections, or disorders of the mouth and oesophagus. In HIV and AIDS infection the gastrointestinal tract is affected by opportunistic infections, which can result in malabsorption and thus weight loss. The patient also has increased nutritional needs because of body tissue degradation from high fevers and opportunistic infections.

Malnutrition results in a poor prognosis because malnourished patients have increased susceptibility to opportunistic infections that can cause diarrhoea, malabsorption, fever and loss of appetite. The result is reduced energy intake and thus a downward cycle.

Individuals with HIV and AIDS infection are often deficient in several micronutrients and are often deficient in B group vitamins. Vitamin B_{12} and vitamin B_6 deficiencies result in mouth sores, glossitis, cheilosis, weakness, mental status changes, loss of appetite and reduced food intake. Fat malabsorption results in a deficiency of fat-soluble vitamins. These include vitamins A, D, E and K. Minerals such as zinc and selenium may also be deficient.

The side effects and food interactions of some of the antiretroviral drugs exacerbate weight loss because these drugs can cause nausea, vomiting, bone marrow suppression, diarrhoea, and glossitis.

There are four main goals that need to be met in order to maintain the nutritional status of the HIV and AIDS patient. Firstly, preserve the patient's initial nutritional status if this is already good. This can be achieved by increasing the intake of nutritious food by increasing the patient's appetite and including body-building foods, energy foods and protective foods. The second goal is to prevent micronutrient and macronutrient deficiencies, which result in a poor immune system. The third goal is to reduce the complications that interfere with nutrient intake and absorption. The final goal is to improve quality of life by preventing malnutrition.

Eating to improve immune function can be achieved through applying the following guidelines. The HIV and AIDS patient needs to eat more fruit and vegetables. Vegetables should be lightly steamed or boiled in order to obtain the highest nutritional value from them. Complex carbohydrates have a high nutritional value and maintain a constant blood sugar level. The patient should eat less fried foods, refined foods and spicy foods. Avoid caffeine because it is an appetite suppressant.

Malabsorption should be addressed early. Malabsorption can be recognised through the following symptoms: diarrhoea and reduced transit time; loss of lean body mass, and foul-smelling and floating stools. Suggest that the patient takes smaller and more frequent meals of high quality. Meals should consist of complex carbohydrates, fruits, vegetables and protein. Fat and diary products should be eaten, but in relatively small amounts. The meals should be simple. Avoid heavy sauces, spices and flavouring. However, the food should still be appealing to encourage the patient to eat. Studies have shown that amino acid supplements may be beneficial. Essential fatty acids such as those obtained in fish oils, flax seed oils and seed oils may also benefit the absorption of vital vitamins.

Decreased appetite is a common problem among HIV and AIDS patients. It is important to isolate the cause of decreased appetite. The following are possible causes: nausea as a result of antiretroviral therapy, depression and despondency, weakness as a result of opportunistic infection, nausea and vomiting, lack of finances to provide nutritious food and dietary restrictions due to antiretroviral treatment or malabsorption. Food should be made presentable and tasty. Allow the patient to select their own food. Exercise is beneficial as this will increase appetite and may improve mood, increase CD4 count and increase resistance to infection.

Nutrition for HIV and AIDS patients:

- The nutritional needs of the HIV and AIDS patient are very important and are greater than normal. Malabsorption, muscle wasting and opportunistic infection compound the nutritional problems of HIV infection.

- About two-thirds of the patient's diet should consist of fruit and lightly cooked vegetable. These have a high nutritional value and the vitamins and enzymes they contain have not been denatured. Juiced fruit and vegetables are highly beneficial.

- Cruciferous vegetables should be consumed in large amounts. These include, broccoli, brussels sprouts, cabbage and cauliflower.

- Ensure that the patient does not become dehydrated. Encourage them to drink plenty of clean water or fruit juice, particularly if they are not eating well.

- Encourage the patient to eat onions and garlic daily. Garlic is considered to be a 'natural antibiotic'. However, remember that garlic may interact with some antiretrovirals.

- Encourage the patient to eliminate coffee, diet drinks, foods with additives and colouring, 'junk' foods, processed and refined foods, saturated fats, salt, sugar and sugar-containing foods and white flour or refined carbohydrates from their diet.

- HIV and AIDS patients should be encouraged to increase their consumption of fibre by either taking psyllium husks daily or an unrefined cereal.

- HIV and AIDS patients should avoid food-borne infections by carefully selecting their food.

- Encourage the patient to avoid excessive alcohol, smoking, substance abuse and poor diet.

- Patients should be encouraged to obtain as much fresh air and sunshine as possible. Apart from stimulating the mood and invigorating the soul, sunshine provides an important source of vitamin D.

Vitamins, minerals and other supplements

An abnormal biochemical environment at the cellular level could result from chronic disease and a catabolic state. This abnormal biochemical environment could represent oxidative stress. Oxidation at a cellular level is dangerous as it makes the body more susceptible to cellular injury and even cancer. Oxidative stress may be prevented by using antioxidants. Such substances include selenium and vitamins E and C.

N-Acetyl cysteine (NAC) is thought to reduce inflammatory symptoms in arthritis and other diseases. This substance has been found to be low in HIV-positive individuals. Increasing NAC levels in HIV patients may reduce inflammation and increase life expectancy (*Elion & Cohen 1997*).

Vitamin C is another antioxidant useful in HIV and AIDS management. Increased consumption of vitamin C in HIV and AIDS patients may result in slower disease progression. Vitamin C has been shown to raise intracellular glutathione and NAC in vitro and also to directly inhibit viral replication. However, all the experimentation has thus far been in vitro and there are no clinical trials to assess the benefit or dose of vitamin C required, so the effects on people are unknown (*Piscitelli 2000*).

Vitamin E is an antioxidant. It has been postulated that vitamin E forms the membrane-based element of antioxidant defence.

Beta-carotene and vitamin A are important in immune function. Poor immune function has been associated with vitamin A deficiency. An individual suffering from a chronic viral infection may benefit from vitamin A.

Pycnogenol, or grape seed extract, is a potent antioxidant.

Glutamine is a supplement that has received attention because of its potential benefit for HIV-positive patients, as their glutamine demand may be increased. A glutamine deficiency results in muscle loss and decreased immune function. Phagocytic function is also thought to increase with the intake of glutamine. In addition, colonic tissue is known to utilise glutamine at higher rates in HIV and AIDS patients, possibly relating to delayed colonic mucosal repair and potential malabsorption. Administration of glutamine in postoperative intensive care patients has been shown to improve absorption of nutrients and encourage a speedy recovery (*Elion & Cohen 1997*).

Selenium is an antioxidant and an essential trace element. The effects of selenium are dose related and it is given in doses lower than 200 mg to avoid toxicity. There appears to be a relationship between selenium deficiency and poor immune function. A selenium deficiency commonly manifests as abnormal CD4 cell function and as candidiasis. Selenium is low in patients with malabsorption. Thus, there may be a relationship between selenium deficiency and HIV and AIDS disease progression (*Wilson et al. 2002*).

Zinc, like selenium, is an essential trace element required by the immune system. Low dosages of zinc stimulate the immune system, but high doses of zinc may be immunosuppressive.

The B vitamins play an important role in HIV management. Niacin and vitamin B_6 normalise immune function and lead to greater immune responsiveness. Vitamin B_{12} is important for neural and cognitive function. Vitamin B_{12} may prevent or improve neuropathy. Vitamin B also helps the patient cope better with stress and depression.

Acidophilus is an essential non-pathogenic bacteria that lives in the digestive tract. Acidophilus is vital for digestive function and aids with absorption. HIV and AIDS patients are susceptible to oral and oesophageal candidiasis. Acidophilus may prevent candiasis.

Co-enzyme Q_{10} is a vitamin-like substance. The action of co-enzyme Q_{10} in the body resembles vitamin E. Co-enzyme Q_{10} is also an antioxidant. Co-enzyme Q_{10} plays a critical role in the production of energy in every cell in the body. It aids circulation, stimulates immune function and increases tissue oxygenation. Oily fish, such as salmon and sardines, are rich in co-enzyme Q_{10}. It is also found in beef, peanuts and spinach (*Piscitelli 2000*).

Protein powders can supply the amino acids required by the body in patients who are not eating well. Proteins are necessary for body tissue repair. HIV and AIDS patients tend to be wasted and thus will benefit from a protein powder mixed with water. Vitamin B_6 (50 mg) and vitamin C (100 mg) can be added to the drink to ensure better absorption. Where protein drinks are not appropriate due to financial constraints, protein complementation is suggested.

Colloidal silver is a broad-spectrum antiseptic. It can be consumed orally or applied to skin lesions. It is particularly useful for the management of gastrointestinal infection, urinary tract infections and respiratory tract infections.

Herbal medicine

In a study conducted in 1997 approximately 35% of those infected with HIV were using CAM (*Piscitelli 2000*). The efficacy and safety of antiretroviral therapy are increasing. However, patients are still resorting to CAM. It is a common misconception that CAM, and particularly herbal medicines, are safe. Some are harmless, but there are drug interactions between herbal products and antiretroviral therapy. There is little information about the pharmacokinetics, drug interaction and adverse reactions of most herbal products. HIV and AIDS patients have high expectations of herbal medicines. They believe that herbal medicine will slow the progression of the disease, improve the immune system, reduce antiretroviral toxicity and even provide a cure.

Herbal medicine and antiretroviral therapy

A herbal remedy that is popular among HIV and AIDS patients is St John's Wort. This is used to treat mild to moderate depression and may have an immunomodulatory effect. However, St John's Wort has also been found to reduce the half-life of indinavir by approximately 50% (*Piscitelli 2000*). The concurrent use of St John's Wort and indinavir can result in sub-optimal blood concentrations of indinavir and thus the development of drug resistance and treatment failure (*Piscitelli 2000*). Furthermore, St John's Wort has also been found to reduce the half-life of nevirapine by 20%.

Garlic is another herb that may be used in HIV and AIDS patients. Garlic is said to modulate the immune system and assist in warding off infection. Garlic also helps to prevent cardiac disease by reducing cholesterol levels. Garlic is commonly used in conjunction with antiretroviral therapy such as saquinavir to counteract the lipotrophic effects of the antiretroviral treatment. But, concurrent consumption of large quantities of garlic and saquinavir reduces the half-life of the antiretroviral.

Echinacea is a popular herb used in the management of HIV and AIDS. Echinacea is thought to be beneficial in maintaining immune function. However, long-term usage of this herb may be toxic to the liver. High doses of echinacea taken concurrently with antiretroviral therapy, which may also be toxic to the liver, may exacerbate liver damage.

It is vital to mention at this point that adverse drug interactions between HIV and AIDS drugs and herbs can occur when adequate dosages of the herb are taken. This implies that the herb should be taken concurrently with the HIV and AIDS drug for a minimum of two weeks and in a high dose for an adverse reaction to occur. Drug interactions between antiretroviral therapy and herbs have been demonstrated in animal studies with the following herbs: milk thistle, echinacea, ginseng, melatonin, and ginkgo biloba. These animal experiments are not necessarily good predictors of human reactions but show that herbal medication should be used with caution by patients who are on antiretrovirals (*Piscitelli 2000*).

Healthcare professionals should always ask patients if they are using herbal substances concurrently with antiretroviral therapy because of the possibility of drug interactions. Patients need to be involved in decisions around their treatment regimen and should not feel it necessary to withhold information from healthcare professionals for fear of a negative and judgemental attitude. Disclosure is vital between the patient and healthcare professionals.

Herbal medicine – the side effects

It is commonly assumed that herbal medicine is safe and has no side effects. This assumption is false. Some herbal products can cause gastric irritation, hepatotoxicity and diarrhoea if taken in high doses. According to the Natural Medicines Comprehensive Database the following herbs can cause the above-mentioned side effects: skullcap, saffron, and some Chinese herbs. These side effects are similar to those expected from antiretroviral therapy. A patient taking antiretroviral therapy and herbs concurrently could experience a severe exacerbation of side effects.

Hepatotoxicity of antiretroviral therapies such as nevirapine may be exacerbated by the following herbs: borage, coltsfoot, mistletoe, and skullcap.

Nephrotoxicity of antiretroviral therapy can be exacerbated by: calamus, chaparral, germander, and germanium.

Cardiovascular disease, heart failure and hypertension could be caused through concurrent use of antiretroviral therapy and comfrey or liquorice root.

Herbal medicine and HIV and AIDS management

Herbal medicine, when recommended by a qualified and registered professional, can be beneficial in the management of HIV and AIDS. Refer to Table 7.1 for an overview of the commonly used herbs for the management of HIV and AIDS (*Piscitelli 2000*).

Commonly used herbs for the management of HIV and AIDS

Herb	Use	Precaution
Aloe vera	Inhibits the growth of the virus in vitro Can be applied to wounds and ulcers	Avoid if the patient has diarrhoea Used for the management of gastric irritation (constipation)
Echinacea	Used for the treatment of common mild infections	Hepatotoxicity

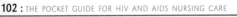

Herb	Use	Precaution
		Allergy
Elderberry	May enhance immune function Treatment of inflammation Is an antioxidant	Hepatotoxicity
Garlic	Prevention of cardiovascular disease May be an immunostimulant Assists digestion Natural antibiotic Can be used in the treatment of candidiasis	Reduces retroviral efficacy
Ginseng	Increases energy Treatment of respiratory infection	
Ginkgo biloba	Improves circulation May improve the blood supply to the brain Treatment of depression Treatment of memory loss	May increase blood pressure
Golden seal	Acts as a natural antibiotic Treatment of oral candidiasis	Should only be used short term
Kava kava	Treatment of anxiety Treatment of insomnia	Can cause drowsiness
Milk thistle	Has hepato-protective effects	
Saw palmetto	Treatment of benign prostatic hypertrophy	
St John's wort	Treatment of depression Inhibits viral infections in vitro	Reduced antiretroviral efficacy Increases skin sensitivity to sunburn

Herb	Use	Precaution
Tea tree	Antiviral and antifungal	Topical irritation For external use only
Valerian	Treatment of anxiety Treatment of insomnia	

Traditional medicine

Traditional medicine is defined by the World Health Organisation as: 'comprising therapeutic practices that have been in existence, often for hundreds of years, before the development and spread of modern scientific medicine and are still with us today. These practices vary widely, in keeping with the social and cultural heritage of the country'.

Some traditional herbs are being studied for use in HIV and AIDS management. These include: *Sutherlandia frutescens* as a possible immune modulator (*Morris 2001*) and Siphonochilus for the treatment of candidiasis.

It is important to consider traditional medicine in the management of HIV in South Africa, as a large proportion of the population relies on traditional healers. Because traditional medicine is part of the traditions and beliefs of much of the South African population, the incorporation of tradition medicine into primary healthcare will encourage people to support community health programmes. Traditional healers are often the first point of contact with HIV and AIDS-infected individuals and thus can play a major role in the prevention and treatment of HIV.

Psychological and spiritual work

Mental and emotional wellbeing is vital for optimum state of physical health, and this is particularly true for individuals with a chronic disease. The new field of psychoneuroimmunology has shown many examples of the way in which thought or mood can modulate immune function. The immune system contains receptors that are sensitive to brain chemicals, such as endorphins, which can modulate lymphocyte and CD4 cell function. Cancer research has demonstrated that maintaining hope and being positive can result in improved health outcomes and certainly in the perception of health. The concept of maintaining hope is central to living with HIV and contributes to resilience and the ability to manage the disease. Patients who continue to find meaning in their lives after a positive HIV diagnosis, by transcending self-image and giving to others, have improved coping abilities and more positive disease outcomes. These patients are also more able to cope with loss and fear.

Chinese medicine

Chinese medicine is an ancient system of healing and can be very useful in the management of HIV and AIDS. Chinese practitioners use acupuncture and herbs. The focus is on restoring balance to the person. Chinese medicine practitioners maintain that the disease process is unique to each individual and so diagnosis and treatment are individualised.

Therapeutic activities

Massage therapy has many beneficial effects and so has become popular in HIV and AIDS treatment. Patients say that they feel calmed, soothed and more energetic and this allows them to cope better with other symptoms of HIV and AIDS. No physiological explanation can be found for the benefits of massage, but touch itself may be healing. Other therapeutic activities include: aerobic exercise, support groups, breathing exercises, psychotherapy, visualisation and spiritual activities, and prayer and meditation.

MANAGEMENT OF THE HIV AND AIDS PATIENT WHO CHOOSES CAM AS THEIR TREATMENT OPTION

It is unrealistic to expect HIV and AIDS patients not to use CAM while on antiretroviral therapy. Heath care professionals should develop a trusting and non-judgemental relationship with patients. Such a relationship encourages the patient to confide in the healthcare professional and disclose their CAM usage. These are some suggestions that will help to obtain a history of CAM use by patients (*Piscitelli 2000*).

Perform a complete drug history. Enquire about the patient's use of CAM, this includes: herbs, homeopathy, Chinese medicine, aromatherapy, reflexology, megavitamins and minerals, massage therapies and other dietary supplements.

Collect and record data on CAM use. Record when the patient started and finished using CAM. Establish if there is a relationship between adverse reactions, immune responses or virological responses and the use of alternative therapies.

Listen to your patients and support them in a non-judgemental manner. HIV and AIDS patients can benefit from CAM, but they can also be harmed. It is vital that the healthcare professional has knowledge of the specific CAM used by the patient and knows its benefits, adverse reactions and drug interactions.

Keep abreast with the latest information. The healthcare provider should be a resource to the patient. The clinic should be a place where the patient can receive accurate and unbiased information.

THE NURSE AS THE PATIENT ADVOCATE

Nurses are increasingly recommending CAM in their nursing practice. CAM is generally considered natural, non-invasive and therefore safe. This is incorrect and CAM prescribed by an untrained or unprofessional individual can be harmful.

The nursing profession has established a rigorous educational programme that prepares registered nurses for practice and registration. To be a registered nurse means that an individual has achieved certain levels of competence in well-defined practice areas. Once the initial qualifications have been obtained it is expected that the professional nurse will embark on further studies, postgraduate education or research. Continuous professional development ensures that the nurse maintains continuous safe practice. A nurse who does not maintain the required level of competence and safe practice can be considered negligent. Nursing regulations ensure that the public will not be harmed by unsafe nursing practices.

The status of CAM is unclear. This can be demonstrated by the difficulties in defining CAM. CAM covers a very broad variety of therapies, some of which are more scientific than others. Occasionally the training and registration of CAM practitioners is unclear. A nurse practising CAM is stepping outside her defined scope of practice. It is important to remember that using CAM, like using allopathic medicine, is not without risks. It is also possibile that a patient using natural medicine may stop appropriate medical treatment or suffer the delayed diagnosis or delayed treatment of a medical condition.

CAM can cause adverse effects and herbal treatments can be toxic or contaminated with toxic substances. Serious reactions and even death may occur with incorrectly administered CAM. It is not correct to assume that natural medicines are safe and have few side effects. For example, acupuncture, administered incorrectly can cause a pneumothorax. The acupuncture needles can also transmit blood-borne infections such as hepatitis B and HIV. All CAM should be given by adequately trained practitioners.

There is limited evidence on the clinical effectiveness and the side effects of CAM. Randomised clinical trails have been few. Where clinical studies have been conducted they have often been flawed by poor design, inadequate sample size, poor statistical analysis and lack of follow-up data.

However, regardless of these factors, more and more people are turning to CAM, possibly because they are disillusioned with allopathic medicine. This disillusionment may include dissatisfaction with doctor–patient relationships or dissatisfaction with medicine in general. Declining support for public hospitals and the introduction of managed care in private practice as cost-saving measures can unfortunately reduce the quality of the service. This will exacerbate the trend towards patients using CAM.

Without the kinds of rigorous professional, educational and regulatory mechanisms that exist in nursing, the public cannot be sure that those who provide CAM, and this includes nurses, have the level of competence to safely deliver the therapy. Nor can they be sure that the therapist will abide by a recognised and enforced code of ethics and conduct. Nurses should be familiar with these legal, professional and ethical requirements when suggesting the use of CAM.

The nurse needs to take professional responsibility for his or her practice. This can be achieved in the following manner:

- *Instill a process of quality improvement*. Quality improvement ensures practitioner and product safety and quality. It ensures safe storage and maintenance of supplies and equipment. Quality improvement includes the continual evaluation and improvement of programmes and practices.
- *Ethical and legal consideration should be taken into account at all times*. Informed consent and individual choice are the most important ethical and legal considerations. The nurse should practise only within his/her defined scope of practice and be accountable for his/her actions.
- *Administration issues need to be taken into consideration*. These include policies and protocols, documentation of modality of application and outcome and incident reporting.
- *The nurse should embark on lifelong learning*. Education should be ongoing. The practice should be according to minimum standards and within competencies.
- *Practice should be in keeping with the Nursing Code of Conduct*. Professional standards of care should be maintained at all times. Nursing practice should be within established healthcare guidelines and cultural and traditional practices of the patient should be taken into consideration.

ETHICAL PRINCIPLES AND PATIENTS' RIGHTS

The use of CAM has raised many ethical issues. Freedom of choice is one such ethical issue. The HIV and AIDS-infected individual should be free to choose whatever medical treatment they desire. The ethical principle of non-maleficence implies protecting the patient from harm. An untrained natural therapist may inflict harm to the patient.

The HIV and AIDS patient has a *right to choose* a therapist and the right to spend their money on the therapist of their choice. This raises the following question – should the application of public funds and resources be directed by consumer demands or should funds be directed towards practices for which reasonable evidence of effectiveness and safety can be provided?

The principle of *beneficence* implies that the practitioner ought to do good and prevent doing any harm. Beneficence is the duty to help another gain what is of benefit to them. In order to do only good to patients, the training of CAM practitioners, which is currently unrestricted, should be subjected to a formal system of regulation.

CAM should be practised according to the rule of *utility*. The service should be provided to bring out the greatest balance between good and bad. The rule of utility is derived from the principle of beneficence and includes the moral duty to weigh and balance benefits against harm, to increase the benefits and reduce the harm. In keeping with the rule of utility, the following ethical question arises – does the community have the obligation to protect vulnerable citizens from exploitation by practitioners holding uncertain qualifications? These practitioners may apply practices with dubious benefits and unknown risks.

Children are vulnerable citizens as they are not always in the position to make decisions about their healthcare provider and to protect themselves. Should special measures be introduced to protect children from practices that may lead to their being denied conventional treatment of known efficacy?

These are all questions that need to be asked when considering patient treatment in general and patient's use of CAM in particular.

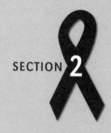

SECTION 2

CHAPTER 8

WOMEN AND HIV AND AIDS

Candice Bodkin

KEY CONCEPTS

- HIV and AIDS and gynaecology
- women and susceptability
- sexually transmitted infections
- contraception
- sexual health
- post exposure prophylaxis
- rape and sexual assault
- prevention of spread of HIV

> The unprecedented rate of new HIV infections among young women in South Africa underscores the feminisation of the HIV epidemic in South Africa
>
> *(Gita Ramjee 2005)*

INTRODUCTION

Women are the group who are most affected by HIV and AIDS in Africa. This chapter will address the physical, socio-cultural, and mental and emotional needs of women. In addition, the factors that increase women's susceptibility to HIV infection will be examined. The role of the nurse in the management of rape and post-exposure prophylaxis will also be addressed.

WOMEN AND HIV

Women in sub-Saharan Africa are at an increased risk of contracting HIV. This is clearly demonstrated by the fact that there are more women infected by HIV than there are men infected in all the sub-Saharan African countries. There are many factors that contribute to the increased risk of HIV transmission in women. These include: social and cultural factors, anatomical factors, the incidence of sexually transmitted infections (STIs), specific sexual practices, and HIV-related factors in the sexual partner.

Social and economic factors

The low socio-economic status of sub-Saharan women is a significant contributing factor to their high incidence of HIV. Low socio-economic status may result in a reduced decision-making ability, which is particularly important in decisions around sexual practices. The incidence of marital abuse is highest among the unemployed and those of poor economic status. An unemployed and dependant woman fears abandonment or even violence from the male partner, and this results in reduced control over practices such as condom use. Women who lack education usually lack knowledge about their reproductive system and thus may lack knowledge about the modes of transmission of HIV and how to prevent its transmission. Society's failure to accept a woman's right to equal access to education and employment reinforces women's dependence on men (*Wilson et al. 2002*).

Poor socio-economic status further contributes to the spread of HIV infection as young socio-economically deprived women depend on an older male partner who offers gifts for sex. The prevalence of HIV is higher among older men, therefore increasing a young woman's risk of infection.

Anatomical factors

Women are the receptive partner in sexual intercourse. As a result, women have a longer exposure to the HI virus in the seminal fluid and have a larger exposed surface area in contact with the HI virus. Furthermore, seminal fluid contains a higher concentration of the HI virus than do vaginal secretions. The vaginal cells also carry receptors that facilitate the entrance of the HI virus.

The early onset of sexual intercourse among young girls places them at an increased risk of transmission of HIV. This is because the lining of the cervix is immature and does not provide an adequate protective barrier. In addition, the genital tract is small, immature and produces scant vaginal secretions. All these factors place a young girl at increased risk of trauma during intercourse and thus at increased risk of HIV transmission.

Rough intercourse and rape cause trauma to the female genital tract. This trauma provides easier than normal entry for the HI virus. Trauma caused by female genital mutilation also increases the risk of HIV transmission.

Recent studies have suggested that uncircumcised men are more likely to transmit and acquire HIV than those who are circumcised.

Sexually transmitted infections

Sexually transmitted infections increase the risk of HIV transmission, particularly if they are left untreated. The stigma attached to STIs makes women reluctant to present at clinics for treatment. Women describe healthcare personnel at STI clinics as being unsympathetic, judgemental and unprepared to diagnose and treat them. STIs also remain untreated because of lack of access to clinics and poor availability of clinics, particularly in rural areas. Many STIs in women may be asymptomatic and therefore remain untreated.

If a woman does have symptoms of a vaginal infection, she may not seek medical attention, as women are socialised to accept ill-health and 'women's troubles' as the norm. Genital ulcers pose a particular risk in the transmission of HIV, because of the large area of damaged mucosa.

Sexual practices

Many sexual practices place women at an increased risk of being infected with HIV, for example, dry sex. Dry sex may be induced through the use of mechanical and herbal substances. Dry sex results in an increased risk of trauma to the genital tract and a subsequently increased risk of HIV transmission.

HIV-related factors in the sexual partner

HIV is more likely to be transmitted by a partner who has an AIDS-defining illness, or who has a low CD4 count or a high viral load. The partner may have a high viral load because they have only recently sero-converted, have advanced HIV infection or have experienced antiretroviral treatment failure.

GYNAECOLOGY AND HIV AND AIDS

Cancer of the cervix and HIV and AIDS

Cancer of the cervix is more common among women infected with HIV, progresses more rapidly and occurs at a younger age. The risk factors for the development of cancer of the cervix and HIV infection are similar. These include: early onset of sexual intercourse, multiple sexual partners, untreated STIs, excessive use of alcohol and substance abuse and failure to use a reliable barrier method of contraception. Furthermore, women who receive treatment for cancer of the cervix have an increased risk of the cancer recurring if they are HIV-positive. Women infected with HIV should have an annual PAP smear.

Gynaecological problems and HIV and AIDS

HIV-positive women experience numerous gynaecological problems, for example, vaginal infections, such as vaginal candidiasis, which may become refractory to treatment in advanced HIV infection. Infections such as syphilis, chlamydia, gonorrhoea, bacterial vaginitis, trichomoniasis and genital herpes are also common in women infected with HIV. All these infections place the woman at an increased risk of transmitting HIV infection or acquiring another strain of HIV infection. If untreated, vaginal infections could result in pelvic inflammatory disease. Pelvic inflammatory disease is usually more severe in HIV-infected women and is more difficult to treat and can result in infertility.

Menstrual disorders are more common in HIV-positive women. Generally, menstrual disorders – particularly amenorrhoea – are associated with weight loss and progressive disease.

Contraception and HIV-positive women

HIV-positive women should be encouraged to use an effective method of contraception.

Sterilisation. It is not unusual for HIV-positive women to plan a pregnancy. With the use of antiretroviral therapy, elective Caesarean section and replacement feeding it is possible for an HIV-positive women to deliver an HIV negative baby. Sterilisation should never be forced on a young nulliparous HIV-positive woman. However, this option should be offered to a woman who has completed her family. Remind the patient that firstly, sterilisation is not easily reversible and secondly, sterilisation does not offer protection against the transmission of HIV. If an HIV-positive woman has been sterilised she should still use a barrier method of contraception.

Intra-uterine contraceptive device. The IUCD is not advised in HIV-positive women because it makes the woman more susceptible to genital tract infections and pelvic inflammatory disease.

Injectable contraceptives. The progesterone only injectable contraceptive is recommended for use in HIV-positive women. This method of contraception is effective and does not result in drug interactions with antiretroviral therapy. However, the injection does not prevent the transmission of HIV and other STIs; therefore, the HIV-positive woman should also use a barrier method of contraception. Injectable contraceptives are useful for young women or women who are likely to forget to take the oral contraceptive pill. Injectable contraceptives can disrupt the menstrual cycle and can cause dysfunctional uterine bleeding.

Oral contraceptive pill. The oral contraceptive pill is an effective method of contraception for HIV-positive women who are motivated and are unlikely to forget to take their contraceptive pill. However, the oral contraceptive pill may interact with certain antiretroviral medicines. A barrier method of contraception is required in addition to the oral contraceptive pill.

Barrier method. The barrier contraceptive method of choice is the male condom. When used correctly the male condom prevents the transmission of HIV and prevents pregnancy. The female condom is also available. The female condom has the advantage that this method is controlled by the woman and can be inserted prior to intercourse. Although effective, the female condom is not always easily accessible in South Africa.

PREVENTION OF THE SPREAD OF HIV INFECTION IN WOMEN

Fostering the empowerment of women in South Africa is an essential step towards the prevention of the spread of HIV and AIDS and other STIs. As previously discussed, the high rate of HIV infection among women is due to their lack of power and control over their sexual risks. It is thus important for the nurse to create opportunities for empowerment among women. One such opportunity is education. This should ideally include information on the prevention of STIs and the importance of seeking early medical treatment for these. Furthermore, women require education around sexual health, on the normal functioning of their bodies, including normal reproductive function and the prevention of pregnancy, and on the prevention of HIV and AIDS.

Healthcare services need to be user friendly in order to ensure accessibility. These services should appropriately address the healthcare needs of the community at an affordable price. In order to be accessible the clinic should be open at times convenient to women and should have the resources to meet the women's needs.

Nurses should support women's groups and community organisations in condemning child abuse, rape, sexual domination and genital mutilation. Sexual health education offered to girls and women only is inadequate for the prevention of the spread of HIV and AIDS. This education should also address the needs of boys and men. In particular, boys and men should be encouraged to engage in respectful and responsible sexual relationships.

Nurses can help to reinforce women's economic independence. Strengthening existing training opportunities for women can encourage economic independence, which fosters empowerment, decision-making ability and ultimately improved health.

MICROBICIDES FOR THE PREVENTION OF THE SPREAD OF HIV AMONG WOMEN

Given the high prevalence and incidence rates of HIV infection among young South African women it is imperative that a safe and effective women-initiated HIV prevention option is investigated (*Ramjee 2005*).

Microbicides are topical agents that are applied in the vagina prior to sexual intercourse, in an effort to prevent the transmission of HIV. They are similar to a spermicide. Microbicides could also be used as a method of contraception or could be used in addition to another method of contraception.

There are currently no safe and effective anti-HIV microbicides available. However, clinical trials are underway and researchers hope that products will be on the market by 2010.

SEXUAL HEALTH EDUCATION AND THE PREVENTION OF HIV AND AIDS

Sexual health education is important in the prevention of the spread of HIV and AIDS and other STIs. A philosophical approach to sexual health counselling is necessary. There needs to be a clear definition of sexual health in the era of HIV and AIDS as well as the other components of sexual health education. Sexual health education for the prevention of HIV and AIDS is one of the nurse's roles, and he/she needs clear guidelines for such education, which will depend on the age of the audience.

Philosophy of sexual health education

The approach outlined below is the author's and can be adapted where necessary.

Sexual health education should be age appropriate. Sexual health education should be started at an early age and the type of information offered should be appropriate for the age of the specific audience. Start sexual education in pre-school children. At this age children are learning about 'good' and 'bad' touch. This way, children learn early that sexual contact between an adult and a child is not 'good' and should always be reported to a responsible adult. Sexual health education should then continue for schoolgoing children, adolescents, young adults, the middle-aged and the aged.

Sexual health education should be culturally sensitive. In certain cultures discussion of sex is taboo. The nurse needs to be aware of this and to discuss sex sensitively.

Sexual health education should be *respectful of individual choice*. The person providing the education should be non-judgemental. This is particularly difficult if a nurse believes that adolescents should abstain from sexual intercourse until married, but the audience of adolescents is already engaging in premarital sex. Abortion is also a very sensitive issue. Nurses need to respect personal choices. In South Africa, a nurse who does not agree with abortion has a legal obligation to refer the patient to another person who will help them. The nurse is responsible for ensuring that the sexual health decision made is an informed decision.

A sexual health education programme for the prevention of the transmission of HIV and AIDS should emphasise *self-worth and dignity*. The programme should take the approach that a woman's body is sacred and should be treated with respect. When women respect and value their bodies they are less likely to engage in risky sexual behaviour. This concept can be extended further; boys and men should also be taught to respect and value women's bodies.

Peer pressure is a significant contributor to unplanned or unwanted sexual contact among adolescents and young adults. It is important for an adolescent to 'fit in' or be accepted by the group and so they engage in risky behaviours to achieve this. It is thus important to encourage adolescents and young adults to develop *positive life-enhancing relationships with themselves and with others*.

A sexual health education programme should emphasise the *positive, life-enhancing and rewarding aspects of human sexuality*. Sexuality should not be viewed as dirty; discussion regarding sexuality should not be taboo. Such behaviour results in failure to ask questions about human sexuality, a lack of understanding about human reproduction and failure to seek early treatment for STIs.

Sexual health education should apply a philosophy of *non discrimination*. Adolescents do have sex; this cannot be ignored. A nurse who manages the sexual health needs of adolescents should be non-judgemental. These young people will need advice on contraception and on the treatment of STIs. When an adolescent visits a clinic for contraception or for the treatment of an STI, they are taking responsibility for their sexual health and are thus a captive audience for sensitive and non-judgemental sexual health education.

If they are discriminated against, they will not return. Many people think that the aged don't have sexual relationships, but this section of the population have their own unique sexual needs and problems.

Sexual health education should provide *accurate information*. Many nurses were trained prior to the era of HIV and AIDS and their knowledge is outdated. It is the nurse's professional responsibility to ensure that their knowledge is accurate and up-to-date.

Encourage critical thinking about gender roles. Women should be encouraged to become knowledgeable on sexual health issues so that they can make informed decisions about their sexual health. Furthermore, women are encouraged to become self-sustaining so that they can move out of a submissive and disempowered role.

Sexual health education should *address the specific needs of the individuals* receiving the education. Specific needs may be dependent on the age of the audience.

Guiding principles

Sexual health education should be accessible. The education provided should be comprehensive and effective. The nurses providing the sexual health education should be trained and should receive administrative support. A sexual health education programme for the prevention of the transmission of HIV and AIDS requires careful planning, and continuous evaluation and updating.

Definition of sexual health

Sexuality is a normal and life-enhancing process. Open communication is the best way to provide information about HIV and AIDS prevention. Sexual health implies independent, open, honest and autonomous and rewarding relationships. A perception of positive self-worth can contribute in a positive manner towards sexual health. Finally, sexual health education helps men and women to make informed decisions about their sexuality and teaches them to take responsibility for their actions.

Components of sexual health education

Sexual health education aimed at the prevention of the transmission of HIV and AIDS should contain the following components:

- The knowledge provided should be directly relevant to the audience.
- The individual should be encouraged to apply personal values in achieving and maintaining sexual health.

- The individual should be taught how to recognise behaviours and resources that are required to meet their goals.
- The individual should be able to translate knowledge into behaviour.
- The individual who has received sexual health education should be able to share their knowledge with others.
- The sexual health education programme should be able to foster self-esteem and acceptance.
- The individual who has received sexual health education should be able to negotiate and adhere to sexual limit setting.
- Individuals should learn how to evaluate the outcome of their sexual health practice, and should then take responsibility for that outcome.
- Individuals should be able to access the materials and resources required in order to ensure sexual health.

Contents of sexual health education

It is recommended that sexual health education for the prevention of HIV and AIDS should address the following issues:

Prevention of sexual abuse

Education on the prevention of sexual abuse should be started as early as possible. The pre-school child is susceptible to sexual abuse and so needs to know what constitutes sexual abuse. Pre-school children should be taught the difference between 'good' or appropriate touch and 'bad' or inappropriate touch.

Psychological, emotional and physical development

Education on development should start during childhood and adolescence. Children need to know about the physical changes that will occur in their bodies as they become sexually mature. This should be taught in a sensitive manner, so that children are not fearful or ashamed of the physical changes that will occur. When providing sex education to children the educator should take psycho-social theories and other developmental theories related to development into consideration. Such theories include: Kohlberg's theory of moral development and Eriksson's theories on psycho-social development. Eriksson's theories address issues such as social acceptance or rejection; identity verses role confusion and intimacy verses isolation, which are relevant to sexual health.

Specific sexual health issues

Sexual health education should include accurate information about contraception and prevention of the transmission of HIV and other STIs. Issues around dating and developing sexual relationships should be discussed. Girls and women in particular require information on the prevention and management of sexual assault. Alcohol and drugs can result in indiscriminate sexual behaviour and so contribute to the spread of HIV and other STIs and their use should be addressed in sexual health education. Finally, contact numbers for support structures, resource persons and local clinics should be provided.

RAPE AND HIV AND AIDS

Rape is a common crime in South Africa and is often not reported because the woman feels humiliated or thinks that nothing will come of the report. Rape causes trauma to the genital tract and thus provides an easy access point for the HI virus. As the nurse is often the first contact for a woman who has been raped, he or she should know how to manage rape and how to prevent HIV in someone who has been raped.

The nursing management of rape

Rape is an extremely traumatic experience. Women who have been raped should be managed with care, sensitivity and empathy. The nurse has three important functions when managing a woman who has been raped. The first is the provision of psychological and emotional support. Secondly, the nurse needs to be an advocate for the patient. As rape could lead to litigation, the nurse should protect the rights of the woman and ensure that all legal requirements are met. Thirdly, the nurse is the woman's healthcare provider. This involves the prevention of STIs and HIV and AIDS, prevention of unwanted pregnancy and treatment of injury.

When the patient arrives at the clinic or hospital she needs to be comforted and reassured and any serious injuries should be treated immediately. She should be taken to a private room where she will be examined by a doctor who is trained to examine rape survivors. Consent must be obtained prior to the examination. The physical examination is very important as this is where evidence of the rape is collected for use in court. The physical examination is also conducted to determine the extent of the injuries. All documentation relating to the rape is completed in triplicate. One copy is sent to the police station. The second copy remains in the patient's personal file. The person who performed the physical examination keeps the third copy in a safe place. It is important to keep this third copy in case the other copies are misplaced. The examining individual may also use this third copy when they give evidence in court.

Prior to examination a thorough history of the rape is obtained. The date, time and place of the rape are recorded as are the date, time and place of the physical examination. Furthermore the nurse should determine:

- the number of perpetrators involved in the rape
- whether or not the woman was conscious during the rape
- the surface upon which the rape took place – such as on the ground, on a carpet or in a car
- the use of violence during the rape
- whether or not a weapon was used, and if so, what it was and how it was used
- whether or not the weapon was inserted into the anus or vagina.

Ideally the woman should not bath or wash prior to the examination. If she has done so, this should be recorded. In a sensitive manner, determine the type of sexual act performed. Finally, determine whether the woman had consensual intercourse prior to the rape.

The woman is asked to undress slowly on a large linen sheet or on a sheet of brown paper so that any evidence that falls from her clothes or body will fall onto the sheet and can be collected. The sheet should be linen or paper, so that moisture can be absorbed and will not damage the evidence. The sheet must be carefully folded and labelled and should accompany the other evidence. This evidence should once again be stored in a paper bag.

It is important that evidence is collected correctly and accurately, as this evidence may be required in court. Evidence collection kits are available, which provide clear instructions on how to collect evidence. For children, a 'teddy bear package' can be used. This evidence collection kit is similar to the adult kit and the same principles of evidence collection apply.

Evidence includes an oral swab, clothing and related items, such as panties or a sanitary towel, and evidence on the body of the woman, including saliva, semen or blood. A swab from under the woman's fingernails, pubic hair combings, an anorectal swab, a genital swab, cervical swab and a reference sample of the woman's DNA are collected. Following the collection of evidence, the woman is examined for injury and is treated accordingly. The injuries should be accurately and carefully recorded, and should include anatomical drawings.

The evidence is locked away a safe place. The police then collect the evidence and the completed documentation. Women are not encouraged to take the evidence to the police themselves in case the evidence is tampered with.

HIV testing is part of the management of a woman who has been raped. This should only be conducted once the woman has given informed consent. She will also be screened for hepatitis B and for syphilis. These initial blood tests serve as a baseline. Should the woman test negative at this initial examination and then tests positive for one or more of these infections at a later stage (six weeks to three months) it is likely that the infection was transmitted during the rape. A pregnancy test is also conducted. If the woman knows the rapist, an HIV test can be requested from the rapist. However, this is often not possible. If the HIV status of the rapist is not known, the rapist is assumed to be HIV-positive and HIV prophylaxis is offered. HIV prophylaxis is also offered if the rapist is tested and found to be HIV-positive. Ideally, HIV prophylaxis should be started within two hours of the rape, but can be started up to 72 hours later. Post-HIV exposure prophylaxis includes zidovudine (AZT) 300 mg administered orally 12 hourly for 28 days and lamivudine 150 mg administered orally 12 hourly for 28 days. It is not advisable that women stop their post-HIV prophylaxis prior to 28 days, as less than 28 days of treatment may be insufficient to prevent HIV infection. A protease inhibitor such as indinavir may be indicated in the event of a high-risk HIV transmission. A high risk of HIV transmission may occur if there is genital trauma during the rape, or where the rapist is known to have a high viral load and a low CD4 count.

The woman should be tested for hepatitis B. Hepatitis B immunoglobulin can be administered to the woman who has been raped to prevent hepatitis B infection.

If the syphilis test is positive the woman requires treatment for syphilis. However, it is unlikely that this infection was transmitted during the rape if the test is immediately positive. Treatment for syphilis includes benzathine penicillin G, 2.4 mega-units and should be given by deep intramuscular injection for three doses, one week apart. If the syphilis test was negative immediately after the rape, the woman does not require treatment, but could still develop syphilis. She should be followed-up after six weeks, three months and six months in order to establish whether she acquired syphilis during the rape. Always enquire about penicillin allergy prior to the administration of a penicillin injection.

If the pregnancy test at the initial physical examination is negative the woman should be offered emergency post-coital contraception. This form of contraception may cause nausea and vomiting, rendering it ineffective. Make sure that an antiemetic is prescribed as well.

The woman who has been raped also requires STI prophylaxis. Non-pregnant women should receive ciprofloxacin, doxycycline and metronidazole. Pregnant women should receive ceftriaxone, erythromycin and metronidazole.

After the examination ensure that the woman can return to a safe place. Assess her need for trauma counselling. The woman may require a sick leave certificate. Ensure that the patient has follow-up appointments booked, and that she understands the importance of the follow-up visits. Examination at the follow-up visits includes assessment of psychological wellbeing, testing for HIV, testing for syphilis, hepatitis B, and pregnancy and asking about signs of other STIs.

It is not only the woman who has been raped who experiences psychological trauma; nurses working with woman who have been raped can also experience psychological trauma and require psychological support and debriefing.

CONCLUSION

Women are the group most affected by HIV and AIDS in Southern Africa. Nursing care must aim to mitigate the effects of the pandemic on this vulnerable group.

HIV AND PREGNANCY

Candice Bodkin

I want people to understand about AIDS - to be careful and respect AIDS - you can't get AIDS if you touch, hug, kiss, hold hands with someone who is infected. Care for us and accept us - we are human beings. We are normal. We have hands. We have feet. We can walk, we can talk, we have needs just like everyone else - don't be afraid of us - we are all the same.

(Nkosi Johnson 2004)

INTRODUCTION

Most children infected with HIV in Africa are infected during pregnancy, labour or breastfeeding. The transmission of HIV from mother-to-child can be prevented through various strategies implemented during pregnancy, labour and infant feeding. Therefore, the management of HIV-positive pregnant women is a vital step in the prevention of spread of HIV.

HIV AND AIDS AND PREGNANCY IN SOUTH AFRICA

HIV and AIDS has been identified as a national health priority since 1994 and is addressed within the National Health Plan for South Africa. The HIV/AIDS/STI Strategic Plan for South Africa (2000-2005) advocates the comprehensive management of HIV and AIDS, the provision of antiretroviral therapy and the prevention of mother-to-child transmission (PMTCT) of HIV.

The provision of antiretroviral treatment is an integral part of the comprehensive management of HIV-positive individuals. Antiretroviral treatment recommended for pregnant women within public sector hospitals in South Africa includes: lamivudine 150 mg twice daily; stavudine 40 mg twice daily; nevirapine 200 mg daily for two weeks and then 200 mg twice daily (*Wilson et al. 2002, DOH 2004*).

Nevirapine (200 mg) administered at the onset of labour for the PMTCT of HIV has been provided to patients in public sector hospitals since March 2002. In August 2003, it was announced that Cabinet was to compile a plan for the roll-out of free antiretroviral treatment for HIV-infected South Africans in public sector hospitals. This started in selected South African public sector hospitals in April 2004.

Free antenatal and intrapartum care is available at all public sector clinics and hospitals to patients without a medical aid. Most deliveries in South Africa are performed within the public sector and are conducted by midwives. Midwives within public sector hospitals in South Africa work either independently of obstetricians or interdependently with them.

The training offered to midwives in South Africa is comprehensive. Assessment and management of HIV-positive pregnant women by midwives include health assessment, screening and referral, therapeutic activities such as the prescription and administration of medication, provision of antenatal care, managing normal vaginal deliveries, and carrying out emergency procedures such as resuscitation, infusion of intravenous fluids and vacuum extraction deliveries. Management also includes the education of the pregnant woman and her family, provision of contraception services, termination of pregnancy services and counselling services.

The escalation of HIV infection in pregnant women now means that midwives provide antenatal care, intrapartum and postnatal care to HIV-positive women and are involved in PMTCT programmes.

TAKING A HISTORY IN AN HIV-POSITIVE PREGNANT WOMAN

The patient history includes the demographic data, medical history, gynaecological history and obstetric history of HIV-positive pregnant women.

The average maternal age of HIV-positive pregnant women

The average age of all pregnant women (HIV-positive and HIV-negative) in a public sector hospital in South Africa is 27 years (*Bodkin 2006*). A study conducted in the USA showed that HIV-positive pregnant women are most likely to be older than 20 years. Maternal deaths due to HIV and AIDS in South Africa are most likely to occur between the ages of 25 to 29 years (*DOH 2002*).

The medical history of the HIV-positive pregnant women

The medical history should include surgical history, pre-existing maternal disease, substance abuse, pica (consumption of substances with no nutrific value) and any maternal risk factors associated with pregnancy.

The surgical history is important because there are certain procedures that make subsequent pregnancies high risk. These are myomectomy, cervical or vaginal surgery, hysterotomy, laparotomy for ectopic pregnancy or for other reasons, and thyroidectomy.

HIV infection is an added burden to the woman's body in pregnancy and results in an increased risk of poor pregnancy outcome (*Ellis et al. 2002*). The increased risk posed by HIV infection is exacerbated in the presence of pre-existing maternal disease. The older the pregnant woman and the higher the parity, the higher the death rate due to pre-existing maternal disease. Pre-existing maternal diseases that are significant in South Africa are cardiac disease, hypertension and tuberculosis.

In South Africa, 0.65% of pregnant women have cardiac disease, which results in a maternal morbidity and mortality rate of 9.5% (*Naidoo et al. 2002*). Cardiac disease in pregnancy accounts for 43.3% of maternal deaths due to pre-existing maternal disease. Undiagnosed cardiac disease (15.1%) and rheumatic heart disease (9.4%) account for most of the mortality due to cardiac disease (*DOH 2002*). Lack of adequate antenatal care has been implicated as a contributing factor to the high death rate due to cardiac disease in pregnancy in South Africa. Apart from cardiac disease, hypertension in the pregnant woman is likely to result in adverse pregnancy outcomes (*Ellis et al. 2002*).

Hypertensive disorders of pregnancy are a major cause of maternal and perinatal morbidity and mortality in South Africa and these disorders should be taken into consideration during the antenatal management of the HIV-positive pregnant woman. Hypertensive disorders in pregnancy include chronic hypertension, pregnancy-induced hypertension and eclampsia. The most common causes of death due to hypertension in pregnancy are eclampsia, HELLP syndrome and liver rupture (*DOH 2002*). Hypertension, like HIV in pregnancy, results in preterm labour (34%), low birth weight (19.9%), intra-uterine growth retardation (6.6%) and neonatal deaths (3.8%).

Tuberculosis is also a pre-existing maternal disease that is significant in South Africa. HIV-positive pregnant women are particularly at risk of contracting tuberculosis, because of the combined immunosuppression of HIV infection and that due to pregnancy itself.

Substance abuse may further complicate HIV infection in pregnancy. This includes alcohol, cigarette smoking and the use of illegal drugs, such as heroin, cocaine and marijuana. Alcohol and illegal drug use have been associated with inconsistent condom use, resulting in an increased risk of transmission of HIV and unplanned pregnancy (*Wilson et al. 2002*). In addition, prenatal exposure to alcohol, cigarette smoking and cocaine could result in decreased birth weight and decreased birth length. Prenatal alcohol use also results in foetal alcohol syndrome (FAS), which is one of the most prevalent genetic conditions in South Africa, along with Down's syndrome, and neural tube defects (*Ehlers 2002*). In addition to FAS, HIV-positive mothers with growth-delayed infants are more likely to have smoked cigarettes or used illegal drugs during their pregnancy.

Pica, also known as geophagy, is the practice of eating soil or clay and is uniquely associated with pregnancy. Pica is thought to arise as a result of mineral deficiencies, particularly calcium. Some African populations view pica as nutritional supplementation and also as soothing gastrointestinal disturbances, particularly diarrhoea and morning sickness. Apart from indicating nutritional deficiencies, eating soil can place pregnant women at risk of contracting *Toxocara canis*, which causes toxacariasis and *Ascaris lumbricoides*, which causes a round worm infestation and *Schistosoma mansoni*, which causes bilharzia. These diseases are particularly problematic in HIV.

Maternal risk posed by HIV in pregnancy

Maternal risk is determined at the onset of antenatal care and pregnant women are classified as normal to high risk. Pregnant women classified as normal risk include those with no risk factors. Pregnant women classified as moderate risk include the early primigravida (maternal age of 15 years or less), elderly primigravida (maternal age of 35 years or more), grandmultipara (parity of five or more), one previous caesarean section, one previous forceps or vacuum delivery, and a history of a previous postpartum haemorrhage requiring a blood transfusion. High-risk pregnant women are those with serious pre-existing maternal disease or maternal morbidity.

High-risk pregnancies at antenatal booking

Previous infertility treatment	Symptomatic asthma
Previous myomectomy	Epilepsy
Previous cervical or vaginal surgery	Active tuberculosis
Previous hysterotomy	Heart disease
Previous perinatal death	Autoimmune disease
Previous baby with major congenital defects	History of venous thrombosis
Last pregnancy preterm at 28 weeks or less	Psychiatric history
Pre-eclampsia in the last pregnancy at 28 weeks	Thyroid disease or thyroidectomy
Three or more previous miscarriages	Deformity of the spine, hips or pelvis
Diabetes mellitus Chronic hypertension or renal disease	Any other serious medical condition

The risk classification can change during pregnancy if any of these conditions occur.

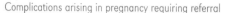

Complications arising in pregnancy requiring referral

Table 9.2		
Anaemia	No maternal weight gain
Uterus large for dates (twins or hydramnios)	Pregnancy reached 42 weeks
Uterus small for dates (IUGR)	Reduced foetal movement after 28 weeks
Malpresentation after 34 weeks	Hypertension and pre-eclampsia
Rhesus negative with antibodies	Antepartum haemorrhage

Source: Department of Health, 2000. Guidelines for Maternity care in South Africa.

The maternal risk is determined by the gynaecological and obstetrical history.

The gynaecological history of HIV-positive pregnant women

Contraceptive advice should be provided to all pregnant women during the antenatal period and during the postnatal period. The male condom is the most appropriate contraception for women who want to space their children and avoid sexually transmitted infections, including HIV. Oral contraceptives and injectable progesterone contraceptives provide good contraceptive protection, but they do not protect against HIV and STIs. Progesterone injectable contraceptives will not reliably prevent pregnancy when taken in combination with rifampicin, protease inhibitors and non-nucleoside reverse transcriptase inhibitors. The intrauterine contraceptive device (IUCD) should not be used by women with a history of STIs within the previous three months or who are at risk of contracting STIs, as the IUCD may cause pelvic inflammatory disease. Surgical sterilisation provides good contraceptive protection but does not prevent the transmission of HIV or STIs (*Wislon et al. 2002*).

The obstetric history of HIV-positive pregnant women

HIV-positive pregnant women have an increased risk of miscarriage and ectopic pregnancy, particularly if the woman is concurrently infected with an STI or syphilis. The risk of miscarriage is increased in the presence of symptomatic HIV infection.

Abortion and HIV and AIDS

The rate of legal abortion in HIV-positive pregnant women is currently unknown in South Africa. However, HIV infection in pregnancy has been significantly associated with maternal death due to illegal abortion in South Africa. The final cause of death in HIV-positive women presenting with septic abortions is immune failure. HIV testing should be encouraged in women presenting with septic abortions, in order to start antiretroviral therapy as part of the treatment regimen.

Caesarean section or normal vaginal delivery for HIV-positive pregnant women

Caesarean section is the delivery method of choice for HIV-positive pregnant women, because this reduces the rate of MTCT of HIV to between 2%–4% (*DOH 2002*). However, caesarean sections are not freely available in public sector hospitals in South Africa and only carried out when indicated for obstetric reasons. However, there are complications in HIV-positive women after caesarean section. For example, the rate of postoperative endometriosis is higher in HIV-positive women than in HIV-negative pregnant women.

The risk of transmission of HIV during delivery can also be reduced by avoiding unnecessary rupture of membranes, avoiding foetal scalp electrodes and foetal scalp sampling, carefully evaluating the need to use forceps or vacuum delivery, carefully evaluating the need to perform an episiotomy and cleaning the vagina with chlorhexidine when doing vaginal examinations.

Perinatal morbidity and mortality for HIV-positive women

A study conducted on the perinatal morbidity and mortality resulting from HIV infection in pregnancy concluded that there is an increased risk of low-birth-weight infants, prematurity, intra-uterine growth retardation (IUGR) and negative perinatal outcomes among HIV-positive pregnant women (*Ellis et al. 2002*). HIV-positive pregnant women were 1.4 times more likely to die during the perinatal period than those who were HIV-negative.

Factors associated with low birth weight in HIV-positive pregnant woman include: CD4 percentage of <14%, previous history of adverse pregnancy outcome, foetal infection, antepartum haemorrhage and *Trichomonas* infection. Factors associated with preterm birth in HIV-positive pregnant women include: a CD4 percentage of less than 14%, antepartum haemorrhage and previous adverse pregnancy outcome. The delivery of a small-for-gestational-age infant by an HIV-positive mother could be associated with substance abuse in pregnancy, *Trichomonas* infection, previous adverse pregnancy outcome and hypertension (*Stratton et al. 1999*).

HIV infection in pregnancy contributes to the high perinatal mortality rate (PNMR) (40/1000 births) in South Africa (*Pattinson 2000*). The greatest contributors to the PNMR in HIV-positive pregnancies are spontaneous preterm labour and intrapartum asphyxia, which is more likely to occur in the compromised foetus, such as the intra-uterine growth retarded foetus or the small for gestational age foetus.

Of the HIV-positive infants born to HIV-positive mothers, 81% die within two to three years. Death is normally due to sepsis caused by overwhelming bacterial infections and opportunistic infections.

HIV-positive pregnant women are more likely to have a history of perinatal mortality, neonatal mortality and infant mortality.

DIAGNOSTIC TESTING

Antenatal diagnostic testing conducted within public sector tertiary hospitals in Gauteng includes HIV testing, syphilis screening by means of a Rapid Plasma Reagin test (RPR), haemoglobin testing (Hb) and Rhesus factor typing (Rh). These tests are carried out at the booking or first antenatal visit. The Hb test is repeated at 36 weeks. HIV, RPR, Hb and Rh are done on site, and results and treatment are offered to the woman before she leaves the clinic.

HIV testing at antenatal clinics

In 2000 it was estimated that nationally, 24.5% of the women who present at public health facilities and are tested for HIV during pregnancy are HIV positive (*DOH 2000*). The figures for 2004 show a national prevalence of 29.5%. These figures are collected during annual anonymous antenatal surveillance.

The primary objective of perinatal care should be to deliver a healthy baby to a healthy mother and this includes the prevention of infection in both mother and child. This cannot be achieved unless HIV status is known. Pregnancy is the time that women are most likely to find out about their HIV status because they are offered testing at the antenatal clinic. Testing should only be done with consent and with full pre- and post-test counselling. The woman has the right to refuse testing. If the woman tests positive she will have to cope with all the potential problems associated with HIV in pregnancy and the possibility of transmitting the infection to her infant. The woman will need support during this period, because of the fear and confusion associated with a positive HIV test.

However, the benefit of HIV testing during the antenatal period is that the woman will now know her status and can act accordingly. The midwife can use this time to educate the woman about possible opportunistic infections and complications which might arise and reinforce the need to consult the clinic staff immediately should she notice them. Knowledge of HIV status aids decision making regarding the pregnancy, the type of delivery and the puerperium. The HIV-positive woman may even choose to terminate the pregnancy and prevent further pregnancies. Knowledge of HIV status aids decision making about safer sex practices. The mother can also be offered treatment to prevent mother-to-child transmission of HIV.

Conversely, HIV testing during pregnancy can result in serious psychological and emotional problems for the mother and the father. A positive test may even result in disturbances in marital or long-term relationships. Crisis intervention may be needed. This is time consuming and requires skill on the part of the registered nurse. Parents can be offered the choice of termination of pregnancy; this is not an easy decision as it may not be in accordance with the parents' religious beliefs or values. Parents also need to address the possibility of the child being HIV-positive and all that this entails, particularly if antiretroviral therapy is not affordable. The parents also need to consider care of the child should one of them die while the child is young. These decisions often leave the parent with feelings of guilt, sadness and fear.

Women who find they are HIV-positive during pregnancy need appropriate and understandable information regarding their health, the health of the baby, options available for termination, information on the PMTCT programme, the type of delivery available, options for replacement feeding and whether or not to breastfeed. Guidelines for pre-HIV test and post-HIV test counselling aid the registered nurse in providing adequate HIV counselling. These are as follows:

- Establish the mother's level of knowledge about HIV.
- Offer information on how the virus is transmitted.
- Discuss the signs, symptoms and progression of the disease.
- Explain the effect of HIV on pregnancy and possible outcomes.
- Explain the risk of mother-to-child transmission of HIV and the options available to the mother to reduce the risk of transmission of HIV infection.
- Offer termination of pregnancy as an option should the mother be less than 20 weeks pregnant.
- Discuss how the woman may react should she receive a positive result and how she will deal with this reaction.

- Discuss to whom the woman may disclose her HIV status. Include in this discussion how she should disclose and anticipate the reactions of others.

- Partner notification is essential as they also require testing, counselling and possibly treatment, but only if the woman has consented to this.

- Develop a plan that protects the woman's safety, should she experience abuse due to disclosing to her partner.

- Refer to the multidisciplinary team where necessary. Collaboration with the midwife, HIV specialist, obstetrician, social worker and dietician is vital for the holistic care of the HIV-infected pregnant woman. Decisions need to be made regarding placing the woman on antiretroviral treatment.

- Plan implementations and referrals to meet the psychological, emotional, spiritual and physical needs of the woman.

- Discuss the prevention of HIV transmission between partners, through the use of condoms.

- Discuss fertility plans and offer sterilisation should she be HIV positive.

- Provide follow-up care, and address issues raised by the patient.

Syphilis screening at antenatal clinics

The estimated national syphilis infection rate for pregnant women is 3.29%. The rate of syphilis infection is declining in South Africa, probably because of improved case management of syphilis at antenatal clinics (*DOH 2000*).

Syphilis is screened for in pregnancy because it can cause abortion, intrauterine growth retardation, intrauterine death, non-immune hydrops foetalis, preterm labour, congenital syphilis in the newborn and neonatal death. These complications can be prevented if the pregnant woman is treated early in pregnancy. If treatment is delayed until the last four weeks of pregnancy, 15% of babies with congenital syphilis will remain untreated (*Cronje & Grobler 2003*).

The screening test of choice at public sector hospitals in South Africa is the rapid plasma reagent (RPR). This test is inexpensive, can be performed on site and the result is available immediately. A second screening treponemal test is recommended when the RPR is positive, to identify false positive results.

All patients obtaining a positive result for syphilis should be treated, irrespective of the gestational age. The treatment of choice is benzathine penicillin G, 2.4 mega-units, administered by deep intramuscular injections for three doses, given one week apart. Allergy to penicillin should always be eliminated prior to administration of benzathine penicillin.

Haemoglobin testing at antenatal clinic

Haemoglobin testing is necessary in pregnancy for the early diagnosis and treatment of anaemia. Anaemia in pregnancy in South Africa is most frequently attributed to iron deficiency related to nutritional deficiency. Other common causes of anaemia in pregnancy are folate deficiency and vitamin B$_{12}$ deficiency. Nutritional deficiency resulting in anaemia is easily overcome by appropriate supplementation. Hb testing in pregnancy should be done at the first booking antenatal clinic visit and then repeated after 28 weeks, preferably at 36 weeks.

Anaemia in pregnancy is defined as an Hb of less than 10g/dl and a haematocrit of less than 35%. Complications related to anaemia in pregnancy are uncommon, unless the Hb is less than 6g/dl. These include high output cardiac failure, inability to withstand obstetric haemorrhage and infection. Anaemic pregnant women may present with the following signs and symptoms: fatigue, listlessness, shortness of breath, dizziness, and palpitations and reduced effort tolerance.

Treatment of choice for iron deficiency anaemia, following a full blood count, includes iron supplementation. If the haemoglobin is less than 6 g/dl a blood transfusion is considered. Parasitic infection with worms or bilharzia infection should be excluded. In addition to iron supplementation, folic acid should be given as well as dietary advice (*Cronje & Grobler 2003*).

TREATMENT OF THE HIV-POSITIVE PREGNANT WOMAN

Treatment offered to HIV-positive pregnant women includes: nutritional supplementation, medication to address an existing chronic medical condition, antiretroviral therapy and nevirapine for the PMTCT of HIV and prophylaxis for opportunistic infections.

Nutritional supplementation in pregnancy

Nutritional supplements that should be given to all pregnant women and should include: folic acid, 0.8 mg daily or equivalent dose, which should be given in the first 12 weeks of pregnancy and if possible before conception; elemental iron, 60 mg daily, from the 13th week of pregnancy and vitamin C, 350 mg daily. Vitamin B complex and vitamin A are additional supplements that can be offered to the HIV-positive pregnant woman. Multivitamins and vitamin A supplementation were found to improve the pattern of weight gain in HIV-positive pregnant women in North West Africa (*Villamor et al. 2002*). Nutritional supplements can be given in addition to other chronic medicine and antiretroviral therapy.

Chronic medication in pregnancy

Chronic medication is required by high-risk HIV-positive pregnant women for the management of conditions such as cardiac disease, diabetes mellitus, epilepsy, asthma and chronic hypertension. Patients with chronic conditions requiring chronic medication are high risk and should be treated by obstetricians in tertiary hospitals.

Antiretroviral therapy for HIV-positive pregnant women

Pregnant women ideally need antiretroviral therapy for themselves, which will also prevent mother-to-child transmission of HIV and treatment for opportunistic infections as they arise (*Patchen & Beal 2001*). If full antiretroviral therapy is not available, then therapy for preventing mother-to-child transmission is offered. Without this, there is a 30% chance of transmitting HIV from mother-to-child, either via the placenta, during delivery or during breastfeeding.

The risk of transmission depends on various maternal factors. The mother is more likely to transmit the HIV infection to her foetus or infant if is she has an advanced or symptomatic stage of the disease, and if her CD4 count is less than 400 cells/μl. Advanced disease or AIDS can be quantified by means of viral load. A high maternal viral load is significantly associated with mother-to-child transmission of HIV. There is also an increased risk of mother-to-child transmission during amniocentesis and other invasive antenatal procedures. There is also a slight increase in transmission during premature labour, prolonged duration of rupture of membranes and in mothers who have had more than ten lifetime sexual partners.

Certain neonatal characteristics have been associated with increased risk of transmission of HIV. These include small-for-gestational-age infants, (less than 2500 g) and premature infants (less than 37 weeks).

MTCT of HIV can be prevented through the use of antiretroviral therapy. The antiretroviral therapy of choice for PMTCT of HIV includes zidovudine (ZDV or AZT), nevirapine (NVP) and lamivudine (3TC). Antepartum, intrapartum and neonatal treatment with AZT have been found to be successful in the prevention of mother-to-child transmission of HIV. AZT used in combination with replacement feeding reduces the perinatal transmission rate of HIV from approximately 35% to 8% (*Patchen & Beal 2001*). As NVP is the drug of choice in South African public sector tertiary hospitals, this drug will be discussed in detail.

Nevirapine for the prevention of mother-to-child transmission of HIV

Nevirapine is a non-nucleoside reverse transcriptase inhibitor. It is used as a short-term, single-agent treatment for the PMTCT of HIV. NVP is useful for the PMTCT as therapeutic drug levels are reached very rapidly and so reduce the viral load rapidly (within approximately four hours). It is used at the onset of labour.

In a study carried out in Uganda, a single dose of 200 mg of nevirapine given to the mother at the onset of labour and a single dose of 2 mg/kg given to the neonate within 72 hours of birth was found to reduce mother-to-child transmission of HIV infection to 13.1%. This is the protocol used in South Africa. In this study nevirapine was found to be superior to AZT, which reduced transmission of HIV infection to 21.5%. A dose of 600 mg AZT was given at the onset of labour, then 300 mg was given three hourly until delivery. The infant was given 4 mg/kg/day for seven days (*Bartlett & Gallant 2000*).

However, although useful for short-term treatment, monotherapy with NVP causes rapid development of drug resistance. When NVP is used as part of antiretroviral therapy, it must be used in combination with two nucleoside analogues and/or at least one protease inhibitor.

The bioavailability of NVP is 93% and is not altered by food or fasting. The half-life of NVP is 25 to 30 hours. The half-life is increased to 66 hours in pregnancy. NVP is metabolised by cytochrome P450 (3A4) to hydroxylated metabolites that are excreted in the urine (*Bartlett & Gallant 2000*).

The major toxicities of NVP are life-threatening hepatic and cutaneous reactions, which usually occur within the first eight weeks of administration. The cutaneous reaction, Stevenson-Johnson Syndrome, presents as a hypersensitivity reaction, accompanied by fever, rash, arthralgia and myalgia. The contra-indications to NVP include concurrent use with rifampin and ketoconazole. Both these drugs are used frequently in HIV-positive individuals and all HIV-positive pregnant women should, if possible, consult an HIV specialist during their pregnancy.

Should the patient be placed on antiretroviral therapy, she needs regular follow-up and blood chemistry including CD4 count, viral load, liver function tests, full blood count, urea and electrolytes. Patients should be educated on the side effects of antiretroviral therapy. See Chapter 4 for a detailed discussion of antiretroviral therapy and the management of side effects.

Prevention of mother-to-child transmission of HIV

Pharmacotherapy in the form of NVP is used for PMTCT of HIV. However, there are also non-pharmacological ways of reducing the risk of mother-to-child transmission of HIV:

- Avoid trauma to the baby during the delivery. Thus foetal scalp monitoring, forceps deliveries and vacuum deliveries should be avoided as this causes trauma to the foetal scalp.

- Avoid trauma to the vaginal mucosa of the mother. Episiotomy is not recommended.

- Consider an elective caesarean section for women who are likely to require an emergency caesarean section, such as women with cephalo-pelvic disproportion, women who have had a previous caesarean section or who have a malpresentation. Should a caesarean section be performed, give a prophylactic dose of cefoxitin 2 g IV as a single dose to prevent puerperal sepsis.

- Maintain intact membranes for as long as possible during the first stage of labour and avoid surgical induction of labour. Rupture of membranes more than four hours prior to delivery increases the risk of HIV transmission.

- The baby should be bathed in the delivery room with soap and water to remove all amniotic fluid, the vernix and the mother's blood, before giving the baby the vitamin K injection.

Ninety-two percent of HIV transmission occurs in the last eight weeks of pregnancy and during the intrapartum period (*Patchen & Beal 2001*). Hence most PMTCT strategies are directed to this period.

Prevention of opportunistic infections (OIs) in pregnancy

Pregnant women with HIV infection develop opportunistic infections. These may present as weight loss, chronic cough, diarrhoea or other chronic illness. The midwife should perform a general physical examination at the first visit and on subsequent visits and check for oral candidiasis, herpes zoster, tuberculosis and lymphadenopathy. Prophylaxis or treatment for OIs should be started as necessary. The OI for which prophylactic treatment is primarily offered is *Pneumocystis jiroveci* pneumonia. The treatment for this is co-trimoxazole two tablets (single strength) taken Monday to Friday or one (double strength) taken Monday to Friday. All pregnant women with HIV should be screened for tuberculosis.

HIV-positive pregnant women should receive hepatitis B vaccination, and the influenza vaccination at the start of winter. It may also be advisable to offer pregnant HIV-postive women pneumococcal vaccination.

PREGNANCY AND HIV AND AIDS INFECTION

Antenatal clinic booking

South African women receiving antenatal care within public sector hospitals in South Africa book at an antenatal clinic at between three and eight months gestation (*Abrahams et al. 2001*). However, delayed antenatal clinic booking is common in South Africa. Reasons for this inlcude being sent away from an antenatal clinic if the woman has not had a confirmatory pregnancy test prior to trying to book. In addition, women in South Africa often have negative perceptions of antenatal clinics, fearing that they may receive poor care while in labour if they are not booked. Women often do not know the best time to book and multiparous women are more likely to book than women having their first baby. Lack of time to book or attend antenatal clinics is a problem, particularly if employers do not give women time off to attend. Antenatal clinics may not be close to the woman's home, leading to long journeys in the early morning to attend on time. Women may also not realise that antenatal care is needed early in pregnancy. Women need more education about the importance of antenatal care.

Antenatal clinic attendance

Adequate antenatal clinic attendance is necessary in order to ensure a healthy pregnancy and safe delivery. The midwife should examine the antenatal patient once a month until the 28th week, and thereafter at least once a fortnight until the 36th week, then at least once a week until labour starts. This is regarded as adequate antenatal care as defined within the Scope of Practice of a Registered Midwife (SANC R2488) and is linked to improved birth outcomes in HIV-positive pregnant women. If HIV-positive pregnant women receive adequate antenatal care there is a 21% reduction in preterm labour, a 48% reduction in low birth weight and a 43% reduction in small-for-gestational-age babies.

Preterm labour, low-birth-weight infants and small-for-gestational-age infants all contribute to the perinatal mortality rate for Gauteng, which was 32.1/1000 and 40/1000 for South Africa as a whole in 2000 (*Pattison 2001*). Factors such as lack of antenatal care, late initiation of antenatal care and infrequent attendance at antenatal clinics contributed to 35.9% of these perinatal deaths, all factors that can be avoided (*Pattison 2001*).

Maternal weight

Weight loss remains a significant problem among HIV-positive individuals. Weight loss due to HIV progression has been found to increase mortality, accelerate disease progression, and result in loss of muscle protein, which in turn results in loss of strength and functioning.

Ideally a pregnant woman should gain 12.5 kg during pregnancy. A significant amount of this weight gain occurs between the 20th and 40th week of pregnancy, where a pregnant woman is expected to gain 0.5 kg per week. However, a normal pregnancy outcome can be achieved even when minimal maternal weight gain has occurred. So lack of maternal weight gain on its own is not indicative of poor perinatal outcome (*Cronje & Grobler 2003*). The average weight gain for HIV-positive pregnant women in West Africa is 306 g a week in the second trimester and 247 g a week in the third trimester (*Villamor et al. 2002*).

Maternal malnutrition in HIV-positive pregnant women could result from recurrent HIV-related infection, which in turn results in poor perinatal outcome. Recurrent urinary tract infections and recurrent sexually transmitted infections (particularly chlamydia) have being associated with maternal malnutrition resulting in low-birth-weight infants.

Maternal morbidity

HIV and AIDS is an indirect cause of maternal morbidity and is currently the leading cause of maternal death in South Africa. Pregnancy nearly doubles the risk of an HIV-positive pregnant woman dying. HIV in pregnancy exacerbates any problems related to the pregnancy. Pregnancy itself does not appear to affect the course of HIV infection during early asymptomatic disease. However, once HIV has progressed there is an increased risk of developing AIDS as the woman's immune system is further compromised during pregnancy (*DOH 2000*). In 1998, non-pregnancy-related deaths caused by infections (mainly AIDS-related) amounted to 23.0% of all maternal deaths in South Africa, making non-pregnancy-related infections the second leading cause of maternal deaths.

Indirect causes of maternal morbidity and mortality

The increasing prevalence of HIV infection in pregnancy is associated with increased severity of disturbance of vaginal flora, resulting in bacterial vaginitis. Non-pregnancy-related infections are those resulting from HIV and AIDS infection, pneumonia, tuberculosis, appendicitis, urinary tract infection, meningitis and malaria. Maternal deaths related to AIDS infection remain under-reported.

FOETAL AND NEONATAL HISTORY

Foetal and neonatal history should include antenatal foetal growth monitoring, gestational age at the onset of labour, birth weight, intrauterine growth retardation (IUGR) and small-for-gestational-age infants (SGA).

Antenatal foetal growth monitoring

The leading cause of perinatal death in South Africa is low birth weight (18.4%) due to intrauterine growth retardation and preterm labour. Many of these deaths could have been avoided and were caused by inappropriate responses to problems identified during the antenatal period, lack of foetal monitoring and delay in referral (*Pattinson 2001*). Currently there are no data available on whether antenatal foetal monitoring using ultrasonography, non-stress testing or biophysical profile testing is useful in HIV-positive pregnancies.

Preterm labour

Causes of preterm labour include bacterial vaginosis, urinary tract infections, and vaginitis caused by a candidiasis infection (*Kjell et al. 2003, Reid 2002*). Twin pregnancies and substance abuse, unemployment, belonging to a low-income group, and lack of education are associated with increased risk of preterm delivery. These factors are related to poor nutrition, higher rates of IUGR, poor quality and quantity of antenatal care, higher frequency of genital tract infections, physically demanding work during pregnancy and higher levels of adverse psychological factors and violence during pregnancy (*Kjell et al. 2003*). The risk of preterm pregnancy increases in teenage mothers and is significantly increased in teenage mothers in a second pregnancy (*Slattery & Moirrison 2002*). Women with a previous history of preterm labour are also at greater risk of subsequent preterm deliveries, as are pregnant women with cervical incompetence due to cone biopsy and previous induced abortions.

HIV-positive pregnant women deliver significantly earlier than HIV-negative pregnant women (37.9 weeks versus 38.5 weeks). Although significantly earlier, the gestational age at onset of labour was not considered to be preterm. The danger of preterm delivery is the increased risk of mother-to-child transmission of HIV.

Birth weight

HIV-positive pregnant women are significantly more likely than HIV-negative women to have low-birth-weight infants (*Ellis et al. 2002*). Causes of IUGR and subsequent low-birth-weight include malaria infection, particularly in sub-Saharan Africa (*Brabin et al. 2003*). In addition, violence during pregnancy has been implicated as a cause of low birth weight infants and preterm labour (*Butchart & Villaveces 2003*). In HIV infection, low-birth-weight is associated with a CD4 percentage of less than 14%, history of previous adverse pregnancy outcome, antepartum haemorrhage and Trichomonas infection (*Stratton et al. 1999*).

Intrauterine growth retardation and small-for-gestational-age infant

Causes of IUGR and SGA include TORCH infections (*Toxoplasma gondii,* rubella, cytomegalovirus and herpes simplex virus types 1 and 2). Other infections that could cause IUGR and SGA include hepatitis A and B, HIV infection and syphilis infection (*Stratton et al. 1999*), Trichomonas. SGA and IUGR are also caused by less than 100% ideal weight in the mother, congenital birth disorders, chronic maternal hypertension, pre-eclampsia and cardiovascular disease, maternal smoking, drug use and alcohol use during pregnancy, twin pregnancies and a CD4 percentage less than 14%.

Apart from increased risk of transmission of HIV, there is an increased likelihood of neonatal ICU admission for SGA babies as well as increased likelihood of an Apgar score below seven at one minute.

MANAGEMENT OF HIV-POSITIVE PREGNANT WOMEN IN SOUTH AFRICA

The Department of Health attributes the high rate of HIV and AIDS-related maternal morbidity and mortality in South Africa to the absence of accepted and practical guidelines for midwives' antenatal assessment and management of HIV-positive pregnant women. In the absence of guidelines, decisions regarding the assessment and management of pregnant women with HIV and AIDS create stress, uncertainty and loss of morale among midwives. Clinical practice guidelines emphasise attention to the following factors in midwife management of pregnancy: maternal age, anaemia, antenatal clinic attendance, maternal weight, pregnancy induced hypertension, syphilis infection, urinary tract infection, vaginal discharge, HIV-related conditions, preterm delivery, intrauterine growth retardation, and birth weight.

Maternal age

The risks associated with extremes of maternal age are relevent to HIV postitive pregnant women and should be assessed by the midwife.

Anaemia

The haemoglobin of HIV-positive pregnant women has been found to be significantly lower than that for HIV-negative pregnant women, so midwives need to diagnose and manage anaemia in HIV-positive pregnant women. Anaemic women need nutritional supplementation such as folic acid and ferrous sulphate. Anaemia in pregnancy results in a reduced ability to tolerate a postpartum haemorrhage.

Antenatal clinic attendance

HIV-positive pregnant women should be examined once a month until the 28th week, and then at least once a fortnight until the 36th week, and then at least once a week until labour starts. Women should have an average of eight antenatal visits. Women should be encouraged to attend antenatal clinics. Midwives need to acknowledge that antenatal clinic attendance is painful reminder of their HIV-positive status for pregnant women and that pregnant women may have difficulty accepting their status and so may miss antenatal clinic appointments. Discuss reasons why the pregnant woman is not attending an antenatal clinic. Possibilities include domestic violence, abuse, neglect, depression and isolation related to her HIV status. Stress the importance of antenatal attendance. Prevent missed appointments by making integrated appointments, where the woman will have her diagnostic tests, ultrasound and antenatal clinic visit all on the same day. Give the woman a note showing her next antenatal clinic appointment. Follow up reasons for missed antenatal clinic appointments (*Patchen & Beal 2001, Abrahams et al. 2001*).

Maternal weight gain

As HIV-positive pregnant women weigh significantly less than HIV-negative pregnant women (*Bodkin et al. 2006*), midwives need to assess and manage maternal weight and maternal weight gain during pregnancy. Weight loss of 10% of body weight is one of the early signs of AIDS. HIV-positive pregnant women should be provided with nutritional supplementation: folic acid, 0.8 mg daily, in the first 12 weeks of pregnancy; elemental iron, 60 mg daily, from the 13th week of pregnancy; Vitamin C, 350 mg daily; multivitamin complex daily and nutritional advice.

HIV-related conditions

The high prevalence of HIV-related conditions among HIV-positive pregnant women means that midwives need to assess when these women should start prophylaxis or treatment for OIs, or even when the woman should start antiretroviral therapy. A CD4 count of less than 14% is an indicator for poor maternal outcome and for increased risk of mother-to-child transmission of HIV.

Maternal infections

Syphilis, pregnancy-induced hypertension and urinary tract infections are significantly increased in HIV-positive pregnant women when compared with HIV-negative pregnant women (*Bodkin & Bruce 2006*). Significantly more HIV-positive pregnant women present with an abnormal vaginal discharge than do HIV-negative pregnant women. Midwives not only need to do a general physical examination, but should specifically test for syphilis, look for pregnancy-induced hypertension and abnormal vaginal discharge and check for urinary tract infections. Complications arising from urinary tract infections, syphilis and an abnormal vaginal discharge include congenital birth defects, septic abortion, puerperal sepsis, pyelonephritis, chorio-amnionitis, preterm labour and preterm rupture of membranes.

Psychological wellbeing

Midwives need to be aware of the psychological reaction of pregnant women to an HIV-positive diagnosis. This may include depression, anxiety and even suicide. HIV-positive pregnant women often do not report psychological problems.

Neonatal outcome

HIV-positive pregnant women deliver significantly earlier, and deliver neonates weighing significantly less, than HIV-negative pregnant women. In addition, the prevalence of IUGR is significantly increased in HIV-positive pregnant women. As a result, midwives need to look for potential risk factors for low birth weight, IUGR and preterm labour and for potential signs and symptoms of IUGR and preterm labour. Potential risk factors for IUGR, low birth weight and preterm labour include substance abuse in pregnancy, *Trichomonas* infection, previous adverse pregnancy outcome, hypertension, TORCH infections (*Toxoplasma gondii*, rubella, cytomegalovirus and herpes simplex virus types 1 and 2), hepatitis A and B, syphilis infection, maternal weight of less than 100% of ideal, congenital abnormalities, cardiovascular disease, twin pregnancies and CD4 percentage of less than 14%. IUGR, low birth weight and preterm labour contribute toward and increased risk of mother-to-child transmission of HIV.

Preterm labour

If an HIV-positive pregnant woman presents with potential risk factors for preterm delivery or potential signs and symptoms of preterm delivery, the patient must be referred to an obstetrician. This assessment should be conducted at the booking antenatal visit and at subsequent antenatal clinic visits. Preterm delivery is considered as birth before 37 weeks gestational age and increases the risk of HIV transmission and perinatal mortality, and should be prevented.

The general physical health of an HIV-positive pregnant women should be assessed through a general examination. A full physical examination should be done at the first antenatal clinic visit and at subsequent visits. Do the following in HIV-positive pregnant women: urine testing (leukocytes, nitrites, ketones and protein), blood pressure monitoring, assessment of oedema, maternal weight measurement, assessment of pallor, foetal movement, foetal lie, foetal presentation, symphysis fundal height measurement and assessment of general health.

Other factors associated with preterm labour in HIV-positive pregnant women include a CD4 percentage of less than 14%, antepartum haemorrhage, previous adverse pregnancy outcome, genitourinary tract infections, twin pregnancies, substance abuse, intrauterine growth retardation, physically demanding work during pregnancy, teenage pregnancy, previous history of preterm labour, cervical incompetence, previous cone biopsy, previous induced abortion, assisted reproductive techniques, maternal disease or infection and foetal abnormality or infection (*Slattery & Morrison 2002, Reid 2002, Kjell et al. 2003, Butchart & Villaveces 2003*).

Low birth weight

All HIV-positive pregnant women presenting with factors associated with low foetal birth weight should be referred to an obstetrician. This should be done at the first possible opportunity or first contact with the pregnant woman and then at subsequent antenatal clinic visits. Less than 2500 g is considered a low birth weight and this child is at increased risk of HIV transmission and perinatal mortality. So, intrauterine growth retardation resulting in small-for-gestational-age infants should be prevented or diagnosed early (*Patchen & Beal 2001*).

Other factors associated with low birth weight in HIV-positive pregnant woman include: CD4 percentage of less than 14%, previous history of adverse pregnancy outcome, maternal disease, foetal abnormality or infection, antepartum haemorrhage, *Trichomonas* infection, preterm delivery, IUGR, malaria infection, abuse and violence, twin pregnancy, less than 100% ideal body mass and substance abuse (*Butchart & Villaveces 2003*).

Suspect intrauterine growth retardation if the following is found: two successive symphysis fundal measurements below the 10th percentile, any three symphysis fundal measurements below the 10th percentile and three symphysis fundal measurements that form a plateau irrespective of percentile. Should IUGR be suspected, the following investigations are recommended: ascertain whether the gestational age is correctly calculated, check foetal heart by means of cardiotocograph monitoring (CTG), examine the abdomen for other signs and symptoms of IUGR, assess whether the cervix is ripe for induction of labour and conduct a clinical examination of the mother to determine the cause of the IUGR. CTG monitoring is used to detect foetal distress. Foetal distress is diagnosed when an abnormal heart pattern is detected. An abnormal foetal heart pattern is diagnosed as follows: baseline heart rate is less than 120 or more than 160 beats/minute, baseline variability is less than 5 beats per minute, or more than 25 beats per minute and deceleration of the heart rate is present (*Cronje & Grobler 2003*).

STRATEGY FOR ANTENATAL CARE

The management of HIV-positive pregnant women should preferably be conducted by an experienced and trained midwife and an obstetrician who is a specialist in HIV management. Pregnant women who have started antiretroviral therapy should attend antenatal clinic more frequently, as they require monitoring for drug side effects and toxicity. HIV and antiretroviral treatment may negatively affect the growth and development of the baby and neonatal growth must be carefully monitored. Most pregnant women book at antenatal clinics in South Africa at approximately 27 weeks, so this is when antiretroviral treatment therapy is started. Table 9.3 provides an overview of the structure of antenatal care for HIV-positive pregnant women on antiretroviral.

Management of HIV-positive pregnant women on antiretroviral therapy

	Week	Activity	Description	Responsibility
Table 9.3	1	Booking visit	• Routine antenatal clinic booking visit	Midwife
			• Routine pre-HIV-test counselling	Counsellor
			• Routine HIV testing	Nurse

Week	Activity	Description	Responsibility
		• Routine post-HIV-counselling	Counsellor
		IF HIV POSITIVE	
		• Overview of ARV in post-HIV-counselling	Counsellor
		• CD4 count done	
		• If >28 weeks ALT done	Dr/Midwife *
2	First visit	• Routine antenatal full assessment	Dr/Midwife *
		• CD4 count and decision to start ARV	Dr/Midwife *
		• Screening for TB in all HIV-positive women	Dr/Midwife *
		THE FOLLOWING QUALIFY FOR ARV	
		* If CD4<200 and <32 weeks pregnant	
		* If WHO Stage IV and <32 weeks pregnant	
		• Consider women with a CD4<350/ WHO stage III	
		• Complete 'screening and staging form'	Dr/Midwife *
		• Complete 'referral form'	Dr/Midwife *
		(Motivate on referral that pregnant women on ARV requires to be fast tracked at ARV clinic)	
2		• If >28 weeks and ALT normal start ARV	Dr
		• Refer or treat OIs	Dr/Midwife *
		• Prescribe Bactrim for 1 month	Dr
		• Refer for ARV and adherence counselling	Counsellor
		• Make appointment at adult ARV clinic for post-delivery	

Week	Activity	Description	Responsibility
		(to ensure continuity of ARV from antenatal clinic to adult ARV clinic post delivery) • *If the woman has been exposed to NVP in a previous pregnancy, she may obtain NVP* • *If woman has been exposed to another ARV regimen consult ARV clinic on best regimen*	
3	Follow-up ARV	• Complete follow-up form & check adherence • Refer for ARV and adherence counselling	Dr/Midwife * Counsellor
4	Follow-up ARV & ALT	• Complete follow-up form & check adherence • Take blood for ALT	Dr/Midwife * Nurse
5	Follow-up ARV	• Complete follow-up form & check adherence • Check ALT • Repeat Bactrim & ARV prescription	Dr/Midwife * Dr/Midwife * Dr/Midwife *
6	Follow-up ARV & ALT	• Complete follow-up form & check adherence • Take blood for ALT	Dr/Midwife * Nurse
7-9	Antenatal visit	• Routine antenatal care	Dr/Midwife *
10	Follow-up ARV & ALT	• Complete follow-up form & check adherence • Take blood for ALT • Repeat bactrim and ARV prescription	Dr/Midwife * Nurse Dr
12 +	Antenatal visit	• Routine antenatal care	Dr/Midwife *

* Dr/Midwife can perform these tasks, depending on the setting.

CHAPTER 10

PAEDIATRIC HIV AND AIDS MANAGEMENT

Candice Bodkin

KEY CONCEPTS

- diagnosis of HIV and AIDS in children
- antiretroviral therapy for children
- nursing management of children with HIV and AIDS
- AIDS orphans

> Of infants infected with HIV, approximately 15% die within two years of birth, an additional 75% die by age ten, and only 10% live for ten years or longer.
>
> *(Churchyard and Metcalf 2005)*

INTRODUCTION

The treatment of children with HIV infection is a highly specialised field of medicine. Initial and ongoing management of children on antiretroviral therapy should ideally be conducted by a specialist in paediatric HIV medicine. This is not always possible in sub-Saharan Africa. It is the responsibility of the healthcare provider to consult with a paediatric HIV specialist prior to initiation of antiretroviral therapy.

The principles for management of children on antiretroviral therapy are similar to those for adults. However, the dosing regimens are different. This is because dosage is calculated according to body mass and body surface area. In addition, children may grow rapidly after starting antiretrovirals and their drug dosages may require repeated adjustment.

Triple therapy with antiretroviral therapy for infants and children is mandatory for the management of HIV and AIDS. As the HIV viral load is higher in children than that in adults, it may be more difficult to suppress the virus to undetectable levels. The purpose of suppressing viral load to levels that are undetectable is to prevent viral resistance to antiretroviral drugs as well as to improve clinical outcome.

HIV TRANSMISSION IN CHILDREN

Mother-to-child transmission of HIV accounts for by far the majority of paediatric infections. Mother-to-child transmission occurs during pregnancy, labour and during breastfeeding. A small proportion of children are infected with HIV through sexual abuse. An even smaller number may be infected by contaminated needles in clinics and hospitals and through infected breastmilk in hospitals when expressed breastmilk is mistakenly given to the wrong child. These forms of transmission are the probably cause of HIV in children whose parents are both negative.

A small number of children are infected with HIV after a blood transfusion. The risk of HIV infection from a blood transfusion is very low in South Africa, approximately one in 400 000 per year.

DIAGNOSIS OF HIV INFECTION IN CHILDREN

Most children are diagnosed as HIV positive based on the presence of symptomatic HIV disease in a child whose mother has a positive HIV antibody test. A child acquires HIV antibodies from the mother during pregnancy, so antibodies present soon after birth may not be HIV infection. Maternal antibodies may even persist in a child for up to 18 months. Diagnostic tests which use HIV antibodies should not be used on children under a year old.

The RNA PCR (polymerase chain reaction) technique can be used to test for viral RNA in an infant as young as six weeks and is the diagnostic test of choice for children under a year.

HIV testing in children and informed consent

HIV testing can only be conducted on children once the parent(s) or legal guardian has received pre-test counselling and has signed informed consent. Post-test counselling should be offered as soon as the test result is available.

STAGING CHILDREN WITH HIV

Children with HIV and AIDS are staged according to clinical and immunological criteria. It is important to stage children as it assists in treatment decisions and in determining the extent of clinical progression and prognosis. HIV infection manifests differently in children compared with adults. The immunological organs and systems grow and develop in children, but are static in adults. In infants and young children, immunological immaturity and young age are the most important determinants of disease (*Cotton 2005*).

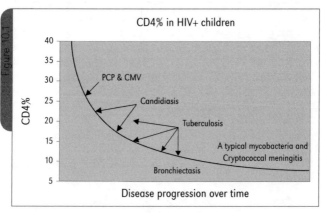

Relationship between CD4 cells, disease and time in children

Source: Cotton M.F. 2005 Classification of HIV disease in children - towards pragmatism? The South African Journal of HIV Medicine November 2005 .

The World Health Organisation Classification system for staging children with HIV infection

The WHO has a four-stage classification system used for the staging of adults with HIV. This staging system was developed in 1994. (The clinical staging system for adults is discussed in detail in Chapter 2). The three-stage paediatric staging system was introduced in 2002. The problem with this three-stage system was that it did not address many conditions seen in HIV-infected infants (*Cotton 2005*). In 2004 a four-stage system for children was introduced.

The revised four-stage WHO clinical staging of HIV for infants and children classify children as follows:

• Stage 1 is asymptomatic.

- Stage 2 includes minor mucocutaneous disorders. Hepatomegaly, hepatosplenomegaly and splenomegaly also belong in Stage 2.
- Stage 3 and Stage 4 include conditions associated with progressive disease.

As with the adult staging system, pulmonary tuberculosis is classified as Stage 3. This is important because infection with pulmonary tuberculosis does not automatically imply that antiretroviral therapy should be started. The WHO recommends that antiretroviral therapy could be started in children presenting with Stage 3 and Stage 4 conditions. A child who is underweight for age is classified as Stage 3 and the marasmic child is classified as Stage 4. Pneumonia is not uncommon in children in sub-Saharan Africa, even among children who are HIV negative, and pneumonia can easily be treated with antibiotics, so pneumonia is classified as a Stage 3 condition. Refer to Table 5.1 for the revised WHO clinical staging of HIV for infants and children.

Revised WHO clinical staging of HIV for infants and children

Stage 1
Asymptomatic
Persistent generalised lymphadenopathy
Hepatosplenomegaly
Stage 2
Recurrent or chronic upper respiratory tract infections (otitis media, otorrhoea, sinusitis)
Papular pruritic eruptions
Seborrhoeic dermatitis
Extensive human papillomavirus infection
Extensive molluscum infection
Herpes zoster
Fungal nail infections
Lineal gingival erythema
Angular cheilitis
Parotid enlargement

Table 10.1

Stage 3

Conditions where a presumptive diagnosis can be made using clinical signs or simple investigations

Unexplained moderate malnutrition not adequately responding to standard treatment (<3rd centile)

Unexplained persistent diarrhoea (14 days or more)

Unexplained persistent fever (intermittent or constant, for longer than one month)

Oral candidiasis (outside the neonatal period)

Oral hairy leukoplakia

Acute necrotising ulcerative gingivitis/peridontitis

Pulmonary tuberculosis

Severe recurrent presumed bacterial pneumonia

Conditions where confirmatory diagnostic testing is necessary

Lymphoid interstitial pneumonitis

Unexplained anaemia (<8g/dl), neutropenia (<1000/mm³), thrombocytopenia (<50 000/ mm³) for more than 1 month

Chronic HIV-associated lung disease including bronchiectasis

Stage 4

Conditions where a presumptive diagnosis can be made using clinical signs or simple investigations

Unexplained severe wasting or severe malnutrition not adequately responding to adequate therapy (<60% of expected body weight)

Pneumocystis pneumonia

Recurrent severe bacterial infections (empyema, pyomyositis, bone or joint infection, meningitis, but excluding pneumonia)

Chronic herpes simplex infection (orolabial or cutaneous or more than one months duration, visceral of any duration)

Extrapulmonary tuberculosis

Kaposi's sarcoma

Oesophageal candidiasis

CNS toxoplasmosis (outside the neonatal period)

HIV encephalopathy

Conditions where confirmatory diagnostic testing is necessary

CMV infection (CMV retinitis or infection of an organ other than the liver, spleen or lymph nodes, onset at age one month or more)

Cryptococcal meningitis (or other extrapulmonary disease)

Any disseminated endemic mycosis (extrapulmonary histoplasmosis, coccidiomycosis, penicilliosis)

Cryptosporidiosis

Isosporiasis

Disseminated non-tuberculous mycobacteria infection

Candida of the trachea, bronchi or lung

Acquired HIV-related rectal fistula

Cerebral or B-cell non-Hodgkin's lymphoma

Progressive multifocal leukoencephalopathy

HIV-related cardiomyopathy or HIV-related nephropathy

Source: Cotton M.F. 2005 The South African Journal of HIV Medicine November 2005(BF3).

HIV occurs as a syndrome and not as a single condition that fits within a single stage. Furthermore, viral load testing is not always available in Africa. Because of this WHO developed criteria for presumptive Stage 4. Ideally antiretroviral therapy should be started at this stage. Refer to Table 10.2 for presumptive Stage 4 HIV infection in infants below 18 months of age where virological confirmation is not possible. Recent research suggests that, in fact, children have the best outcome if antiretroviral therapy is started early in disease. However, this is generally not possible in southern Africa, where resources are poor.

Presumptive Stage 4 HIV infection in infants below 18 months of age where virological confirmation is not possible

Table 10.2

- HIV seropositive infant less than 18 months, symptomatic with two or more of the following: oral thrush, +/- severe pneumonia, +/- severe wasting or malnutrition, +/- severe sepsis, severe immunosupression should commence antiretroviral therapy.

- CD4 values, where available, may be used to guide decision making, CD4 % below 25% requires antiretroviral therapy.

- Other factors that support diagnosis of clinical Stage 4 HIV infection in an HIV-seropositive infant are recent maternal death or advanced HIV disease in the mother.

- Confirmation of HIV diagnosis should be sought as soon as possible.

Source: Cotton N.F. 2005. The South African Journal of HIV Medicine. November 2005

VIRAL LOAD AND CD4 COUNT IN CHILDREN

Viral load

Viral loads are higher in children in their first year of life, relative to adult values. The viral load only declines to adult values at approximately five to six years. By two months of age, HIV-infected infants have, on average, a viral load of 100 000 RNA copies/ml of plasma. The range is from undetectable to 10 million RNA copies/ml of plasma. It is generally accepted that the higher the viral load, the more rapid the disease progression; however, this may be variable.

The measurement of viral load is helpful in monitoring response to antiretroviral therapy. Monitoring of CD4 count is useful in predicting mortality.

CD4 count and CD4 percentage

The CD4 count should be measured whenever the viral load is measured in children. In children, particularly those under two years of age, a CD4 percentage is used to measure immune function rather than the CD4 cell count because CD4 count varies with age in children. A CD4% of 15% can be viewed as similar to a CD4 count of less than 200 cells/μl.

GOALS OF ANTIRETROVIRAL THERAPY IN CHILDREN

The goals of antiretroviral therapy in children are:
- maximal and durable suppression of the viral load
- restoration and preservation of immune function as determined by CD4 count
- reduction in morbidity and mortality
- prevention of opportunistic infections
- treatment of intercurrent infections.

In addition children need nutritional support and general supportive care.

Antiretroviral therapy enhances the quality and quantity of life of HIV-infected children and performs a role in improving the physical, social and intellectual development of the HIV-infected child. Antiretroviral treatment can reduce hospitalisation, because it reduces the incidence of opportunistic infections. Parents are very concerned about the health of their child, when the health of the child is generally good, the mental and emotional wellbeing of the parent is improved (*Cotton 2005*).

ANTIRETROVIRAL THERAPY AND CHILDREN

When to start antiretroviral therapy

Children being considered for antiretroviral therapy will need to meet both medical and psychosocial criteria before starting therapy (*DOH 2004*).

Medical criteria

These are:

* recurrent hospitalisations (>2 admissions per year) for HIV-related disease, or a single prolonged hospitalisation (>4 weeks)
  OR
* modified WHO Stage 2 or Stage 3 disease
  OR
* CD4 percentage <20% in a child under 18 months old, irrespective of disease stage
  OR
* CD4 percentage <15% in a child over 18 months old, irrespective of disease stage.

Psychosocial criteria

These are:

* an identifiable and responsible adult who is able to administer medication
* demonstrated reliability in the adult caregiver
* supportive social environment with adults present in the household
* disclosure to another adult living in the same house.

Pharmacokinetics and pharmacodynamics

The use of antiretroviral therapy in paediatrics requires careful management. The dosages, route of administration, half-life, and distribution of the drugs all differ in the child compared with the adult. Furthermore, paediatric drug regimens need to be altered according to the weight of the child. Initially the child may be underweight as they failed to grow adequately due to recurrent infections. However, once the same child starts antiretroviral therapy they may suddenly grow rapidly as they are no longer plagued by repeated infections. This means that children should be weighed at each clinic visit and if necessary, the dose of their antiretroviral therapy should be adjusted.

Infants have reduced gastric acid and reduced lipase secretion; both affect the absorption of antiretroviral therapy. Furthermore, infants have lower plasma protein concentrations and have a higher body water content, which affects drug distribution and deposition. Drugs are excreted via the kidneys or the liver. Elimination via the kidneys or liver may be reduced in the infant and then increase as the child grows. This needs to be taken into consideration when calculating dosages. Infants in particular may have problems eliminating drugs, so smaller dosages should be administered to them.

Children have difficulty in swallowing tablets, so the antiretroviral therapy should preferably be administered as a liquid. However, many antiretroviral formulations are not available in liquid form, and if they are, may taste very bad and so are difficult to give to a child. Where drugs are not available in liquid form, tablets may be given, but these will need to be crushed, so that they can be swallowed. Crushing or mixing with foods may reduce drug absorption. It is important for the healthcare provider to check how the tablets are being administered to children and to ensure that drug absorption is optimal.

Some liquid formulations of antiretroviral drugs require refrigeration. In South Africa, many households do not have access to refrigerators and so the drugs cannot be safely stored.

ANTIRETROVIRAL REGIMENS IN CHILDREN

The regimens presented are those recommended by the National Department of Health (South Africa) (*DOH 2004*). Children in the private sector should receive the same regimens as those in the public sector to facilitate patient movement between the private and public sector and to prevent the emergence of drug resistance.

Antiretroviral therapy for the paediatric patient

Table 10.3

Drug	Dose	Major toxicities	Other comments
Abacavir (ABC)	*All ages:* 8 mg/kg/dose	Nausea, vomiting, fever, headache, diarrhoea, rash, anorexia, lactic acidosis, hypersensitivity, pancreatitis, hepatitis	Available in syrup and is well tolerated. Where syrup is not available, the tablet may be crushed. Warn the caregiver about hypersensitivity reaction. If hypersensitivity reaction does occur, stop ABC and do not rechallenge.
Didanosine (ddI)	*Neonates:* 50 mg/m^2/ dose BD *Paediatric:* 90–120 mg/m^2 BD	GIT disturbance, peripheral neuropathy, electrolyte disturbance, lactic acidosis, hepatitis, pancreatitis, diarrhoea	The suspension requires refrigeration and should be shaken well before use. Needs to be administered 1 hour before or 2 hours after food. The capsule may be opened and sprinkled on food for children.
Lamivudine (3TC)	*Neonates:* 2 mg/kg BD *Paediatrics:* 4 mg/kg BD	Headache, fatigue, GIT disturbance, pancreatitis, peripheral neuropathy, neutropaenia, lactic acidosis, hepatitis	Can be given with food. The suspension can be kept at room temperature but should be used within one month of opening.

Drug	Dose	Major toxicities	Other comments
Zidovudine (ZDV or AZT)	*Neonate:* 4 mg/kg/dose BD *Paediatrics:* 180–240 mg/m² BD	Anaemia, neutropaenia, headache, myopathy, hepatitis, lactic acidosis	The large volume of syrup required by older children is not well tolerated. Requires storage in a glass bottle and is light sensitive. Can be given with food. Do not use with stavudine as antagonistic.
Stavudine (d4T)	*Neonate:* 0.5 mg/kg/dose BD *Paediatrics* 1 mg/kg/dose BD	Headache, gastrointestinal disturbances, rash, peripheral neuropathy, pancreatitis, lactic acidosis	Suspension requires refrigeration and is stable for 30 days. Requires storage in a glass bottle and to be shaken well before administration. Capsules may be opened and mixed with a small amount of food. Do not use with AZT as is antagonistic.
Efavirenz (EFV)	10-<15 kg: 200 mg 15-<20 kg: 250 mg 20-<25 kg: 300 mg 25-<32.5 kg: 350 mg 32.5 kg-<40 kg: 400 mg	Dizziness, dream and sleep disturbance, agitation, feeling 'disconnected', impaired concentration, hallucinations, rash	Capsules can be opened and mixed with food but have a peppery taste. Avoid administration with a high-fat meal. Administer at bedtime to reduce CNS side

Drug	Dose	Major toxicities	Other comments
	>40 kg: 600 mg Daily dose		effects.
Nevirapine (NVP)	*Neonates:* 5 mg/kg daily for 14 days, then 120 mg/m² / dose BD, for 14 days, then 200 mg/m² /dose BD *Paediatric:* 120–200 mg/m² /dose daily for 14 days then increase to BD	Skin rash (Stevens-Johnson syndrome) fever, nausea, headache, elevated liver enzymes, hepatitis, hypersensitivity	Can be given with food. The suspension can be stored at room temperature. Shake suspension well before use. Warn caregiver about rash and Stevens-Johnson syndrome. If rash does occur and is severe, then stop NVP.
Lopinavir/ ritonavir (LPV/RTV)	*Infants <6 months:* 300 mg/ m² BD	Diarrhoea, headache, nausea, vomiting, hyperlipidaemia, hypercholestero-lemia, hyperglycaemia, ketoacidosis, diabetes, hepatitis	Oral solutions and capsules should be preferably refrigerated, but can be stored at room temperature for up to two months. The liquid formulation contains alcohol and has a bitter taste. Take with food. Has numerous drug interactions.

Source: Patel, Best & Capparelli. 2005. The South African Journal of HIV Medicine. November 2005 .

First-line regimen

Children six months to three years

Stavudine + lamivudine + lopinavir/ritonavir

Children older than three years or >10 kg

Stavudine + lamivudine + efavirenz

Second-line regimen

Children six months to three years

Zidovudine + didanosine + nevirapine/efavirenz

Children older than three years or >10 kg

Zidovudine + didanosine + lopinavir/ritonavir

ANTIRETROVIRAL THERAPY AFTER FAILED PMTCT PROPHYLAXIS

Prevention of mother-to-child transmission of HIV programmes in South Africa involves the administration of a single dose of nevirapine to the mother at the onset of labour and administration of a single dose of nevirapine to the baby within 72 hours of birth. Where this PMTCT prophylaxis fails, it is thought that the child may have developed resistance to nevirapine, and so nevirapine should be avoided in these children in the future. Cross-resistance to efavirenz may also occur in these children, and ideally efavirenz should also be avoided.

INITIATING ANTIRETROVIRAL THERAPY IN CHILDREN

The first visit

An accurate HIV-positive diagnosis should be obtained, following which, the child's stage of HIV infection should be established. The revised WHO clinical staging of HIV for infants and children can be used. Prior to the initiation of antiretroviral therapy, a CD4 percentage and a viral load should be obtained. These values serve as a baseline for monitoring antiretroviral treatment.

Growth monitoring is vital in children. The HIV-positive child requiring antiretroviral therapy is likely to be malnourished and even stunted due to repeated opportunistic infections. Once again a baseline for weight, height and head circumference should be obtained. These are plotted on a growth chart appropriate for the age and sex of the child. This growth monitoring should be conducted at least every visit, as the child may grow more rapidly following the initiation of antiretroviral therapy. In addition, careful and accurate weight monitoring is important in children, because the drug dosages depend on the weight of the child or calculation of body surface area.

As the child may not have received treatment prior to this visit, the child may require a full physical examination to rule out opportunistic infections. These opportunistic infections require treatment before the start of antiretroviral therapy. One such opportunistic infection is pulmonary tuberculosis. The treatment for tuberculosis should ideally be completed prior to the initiation of antiretroviral therapy because children may not be able to tolerate anti-TB drugs as well as antiretroviral therapy.

Adherence counselling should be conducted at each visit, including this first visit. Topics to be covered in adherence counselling at the first visit are:

* HIV prognosis
* antiretroviral treatment
* adherence
* drug formulations
* taste issues, dosage regimens and storage
* opportunistic infection prophylaxis.

The prophylaxis for opportunistic infections issued at this visit can be used to test adherence. The parent, or caregiver of the child should receive clear instructions on how to administer the treatment. When they return to the clinic for the second visit, the healthcare provider can assess whether the parent or caregiver was able to adhere to the treatment regimen. If adherence to the prophylaxis for opportunistic infections was good, it is likely that adherence to the antiretroviral therapy will be good. Refer to the discussion on maintaining adherence in Chapter 4.

At the end of the first consultation, the parent or caregiver should be given the contact details of the treating staff. This is important in the event that the child develops an adverse reaction to the treatment. Ensure that all questions have been answered prior to allowing the parent/caregiver to leave the clinic.

The second visit

The CD4 percentage and viral load results should be available. A final decision on whether or not to start antiretroviral therapy can be made, based on this information. Growth monitoring should be done. If treatment for an infection was administered, this should be followed up. The healthcare provider should also assess adherence to the prophylactic treatment. If the healthcare provider is satisfied that the child meets all the inclusion criteria required to start antiretrovirals and is satisfied that the parents/caregiver are adequately informed, antiretroviral therapy may be started at this visit. Adherence counselling should ideally be repeated at this visit. The parent/caregiver should be reminded of potential adverse reactions and what to do in the event of the child developing adverse reactions.

Clear instructions should be issued on how to take the drugs. The instructions should include graphic instructions, for example a drawing of a moon for the evening dose and a drawing of a rising sun for the morning dose.

Phone call

It is recommended that the healthcare provider phone the family after one week to establish the level of adherence and whether there are any problems with taking the antiretroviral therapy.

The third visit

The third visit should ideally occur two weeks after starting antiretroviral therapy. Adherence is checked and growth monitoring is repeated at this visit. The healthcare provider should pay special attention to adverse reactions, the identification of adverse reactions and the treatment of adverse reactions.

The fourth visit

The fourth visit should take place four weeks after starting antiretroviral therapy. Once again, adherence should be checked and growth monitoring repeated. Safety blood tests can be done at this visit to monitor drug toxicity.

The follow-up visits

The child requires follow-up consultation and repeat prescriptions monthly. These follow-up consultations can be conducted by a nurse, particularly if the clinic is in a rural or poorly serviced area. However, should the child develop any drug toxicities or infections, the child should be referred to the doctor. Growth monitoring, monitoring of adverse reactions and adherence should be done at each visit.

If the child is tolerating the antiretroviral therapy well, the child needs to see the doctor only at three months and then at six months after starting treatment. Blood tests for viral load and CD4 percentage are conducted at the three month and six month visit. If the doctor is satisfied with the progress of the child, children older than two years can be seen by the doctor six monthly and children under two years should be seen by the doctor three monthly.

PROPHYLAXIS FOR OPPORTUNISTIC INFECTIONS

All HIV-infected and HIV-exposed children should receive co-trimoxazole prophylaxis for *Pneumocystis* pneumonia from six weeks of life. This may be stopped if the child is found to be HIV-negative; if the CD4 percentage is more than 20% in a child older than one year; or if the there is immune recovery to a CD4 percentage of more than 20% after starting antiretroviral therapy and the child is older than one year.

TREATMENT FAILURE

Serial viral load and CD4 count or CD4 percentage analysis is used to determine whether treatment is successful. The decision to switch antiretroviral regimens in children should be taken seriously, as there are few regimens available for use in children.

Antiretroviral treatment failure is suspected when the CD4 count or CD4 percentage continues to decline, despite best efforts, including step-up adherence counselling. Treatment failure should also be suspected if there is evidence of clinical deterioration. Such evidence includes:

- growth failure
- neurodevelopmental deterioration
- disease progression (progression from Stage 3 to Stage 4).

Viral load and CD4 testing may be variable, particularly if the child has an intercurrent illness. It is advisable to wait one month after the intercurrent infection has resolved before retesting the viral load and CD4 count. If the CD4 count or CD4 percentage remains low, or the viral load is increased, then a change in antiretroviral regimen may be indicated. The nurse should refer the child to a paediatric HIV specialist for further management.

ANTIRETROVIRAL THERAPY AND ADOLESCENTS

For pre-pubertal and early pubertal adolescents use the paediatric guidelines for antiretroviral administration and management. Post-pubertal adolescents may be managed on antiretroviral therapy according to adult guidelines and regimens.

Adolescents may not adhere well to treatment as their treatment may not be managed by a parent or caregiver. However, adolescents may respond well to positive reinforcement. During this stage of life, the healthcare provider should encourage responsibility and acknowledge that adolescents need to take responsibility for their own treatment. In order to overcome poor adherence the healthcare provider should provide clear instructions, apply step-up adherence strategies and recommend an increased frequency of visits.

CONCOMITANT TUBERCULOSIS IN CHILDREN

Tuberculosis is a common co-morbid condition in children with HIV and AIDS. There are two treatment scenarios to consider when treating HIV-positive children for TB.

The child presents with tuberculosis before starting antiretroviral therapy

- Complete TB treatment before commencing antiretroviral therapy, or at least complete two months of TB treatment before commencing antiretrovirals.
- If the child has failed the nevirapine vertical transmission programme, or is less than three years old or weighs less than 10 kg, use ritonavir as the third drug.
- If the child was not on the nevirapine vertical transmission programme, is more than three years old and weighs more than 10 kg, use efavirenz as the third drug.
- Monitor liver enzymes (ALT) monthly for the first six months of antiretroviral therapy and then as clinically indicated.

The child develops tuberculosis while on antiretroviral therapy

- If the child is on lopinavir/ritonavir, then switch to ritonavir.
- If the child is on nevirapine, is less than three years old and weighs less than 10 kg, switch the nevirapine to ritonavir.

- If the child is on nevirapine, is more than three years old and weighs more than 10 kg, switch the nevirapine to efavirenz.
- If the child is unable to tolerate anti-TB drugs as well as antiretroviral therapy, the antiretroviral therapy should be stopped for the duration of the TB treatment. On completion of TB treatment, antiretroviral therapy may be resumed.
- Monitor liver enzymes (ALT) monthly for the first six months of antiretroviral therapy and then as clinically indicated.

TB TREATMENT AND ANTIRETROVIRAL THERAPY IN CHILDREN

There are numerous drug interactions between TB treatment and antiretroviral therapy, particularly the NNRTIs and PIs. As a result the TB treatment or antiretrovirals or both need to be adjusted. Furthermore, children have difficulties in tolerating the high tablet load and drug toxicities of combined anti-TB treatment and antiretroviral therapy.

The ideal scenario would be to delay antiretroviral therapy until TB treatment is complete. Furthermore, allow two weeks after the completion of TB treatment for the liver to clear rifampicin prior to starting antiretroviral therapy.

If the CD4 count is low and the child should commence antiretroviral treatment according to treatment guidelines, then wait one to two months after starting TB treatment before starting antiretrovirals.

TO BREASTFEED OR TO GIVE THE BOTTLE?

The issue of infant feeding in South Africa is very controversial. 'Breast is best' but breastfeeding results in the transmission of HIV from mother to child. 'Bottle is best' in the prevention of mother-to-child transmission of HIV, but bottle-feeding is associated with high cost and a high infant mortality due to gastrointestinal infections.

The establishment of infant feeding practices, as described in the 'Protocol for providing a comprehensive package of care for the prevention of mother-to-child transmission of HIV in South Africa' suggests the following with respect to infant feeding. *'In an ideal world where safe and adequate formula feeding is possible, and where ongoing support for mother and monitoring of an infant are available, formula feeding is the principle recommended method of feeding. The risk of feeding an infant with replacement formula must be balanced against the risks of HIV transmission through breastfeeding.'*

The protocol goes on to state that it is important not to be dogmatic in one's approach towards either one or the other option. It is advisable to assess every HIV-positive mother individually, and to assess the risk posed in each individual instance prior to making a suggestion on which feeding option is best. It is important to let the patient have a say in her choice of infant feeding.

Women who opt for breastfeeding require counselling and support so that they understand that they must exclusively breastfeed their baby and not provide any supplemental feeding, not even water. Good breastfeeding techniques and hygiene are necessary to reduce the risk of mother-to-child transmission of HIV.

In the event that a woman chooses to bottle feed her infant she should be supplied with the correct information and educational material to ensure proper infant formula feeding. The information should include the social and financial implications of formula feeding. Mothers should be informed of the health hazards accompanying the use of formula feeding. Prior to a mother being discharged from hospital with her newborn baby, she should have received a comprehensive demonstration on all practical aspects of formula feeding.

Antenatal discussion on infant feeding should include the following:

- the risk of HIV transmission through breastfeeding
- the benefits of breastfeeding
- the risks of mixed feeding
- formula feeding can be recommended where:
  - clean and safe water is available
  - equipment and utensils for safe preparation of formula are available
  - safe administration of formula through a cup or sterilised bottle is available
- feasibility and acceptability of exclusive breastfeeding or feasibility and acceptability of exclusive formula feeding.

Postnatal advice for women choosing to exclusively formula feed their infants:

- correct and safe preparation of feeding
- benefits of cup feeding
- demonstration of preparation of a bottle and bottle-feeding prior to discharge from hospital.

Give the mother a pamphlet on safe formula feeding. Free commercial formula should be issued on discharge to last at least two weeks (this is available at most South African public sector hospitals and clinics). Mothers choosing to formula feed their infants should receive formula from their local clinic for at least six months after birth.

Postnatal advice for women choosing to exclusively breastfeed their infants:

- Special attention should be paid to attachment and positioning of the infant on the breast.
- Provide strategies to prevent and manage sore and cracked nipples, engorged breasts and mastitis.
- Recommend exclusive breastfeeding day and night on demand for at least for four months.
- The baby should be weaned off the breast abruptly at four months.
- After four months the mother will be provided with formula for two months, until the baby is six months old.

AIDS ORPHANS IN SOUTH AFRICA

A baby born to an HIV-positive mother has close to a 100% chance of being orphaned before reaching the age of ten. In South Africa, nearly one million children under the age of 15 had lost their mothers to HIV by 2005 (*Whiteside 2000*). Furthermore, in the absence of widespread antiretroviral treatment, an estimated four million children, or about 10% of the entire South African population, will be orphaned by the year 2015 (*Madhavan 2004*). Orphans are less likely to receive adequate parenting, education, and nutrition. Orphans may land up on the streets and thus will be more likely to face sexual abuse and exploitation and so be at risk of HIV infection themselves. The orphans that AIDS is creating pose serious social, economic, political, and developmental challenges for South Africa.

Problems faced by orphans

The problems faced by orphans may have begun prior to the death of their parents. These children may have had to take on adult roles and nurse sick parents who were dying from AIDS. These often very young children may have watched their parent/parents die. Whilst nursing the sick parent/s the child may not have been told the cause of the parent's illness. These children may only find out later that their parent died of AIDS, or may never know why their parent died.

Following the death of the parent the child may experience guilt, depression and post-traumatic disorder. These psychological and emotional problems may have long-term consequences.

The newly orphaned child may face discrimination by members of the local community. These children may even be exploited by the extended family. Orphans may need to stay in their family home to ensure that they inherit the property.

Generally the oldest child becomes the breadwinner. This child may have to leave school and start work in order to provide for younger siblings. The household becomes a child-headed household. The fact that the eldest child has to drop out of school means that this child does not receive education and this perpetuates the cycle of poverty.

Many orphans in child-headed households live below the breadline. These orphans do not have any food security and often do not eat for days. Lack of food security results in malnutrition. A malnourished child is more susceptible to infectious diseases. Furthermore, a malnourished child is unable to perform at school; this may result in low self-esteem and high drop-out rates.

Care of orphans in South Africa

Options for alternative means of care for AIDS orphans include:

* accommodation with extended families
* accommodation with foster care families within the community
* accommodation with a group of paid foster care mothers within the community
* adoption
* day care/orphan centres
* children's homes.

The ideal would be to accommodate orphans in the homes of extended families. However, as the number of orphans increase, the resources of already poor communities are further strained and this may not be possible. Strategies need to be developed to support the extended families or to support orphans in the absence of extended families.

Over the past few years there has been an increase in the availability of grants for orphaned children and their carers. There are also many public-private partnerships in which large companies are providing the finance necessary to support AIDS orphans in their communities. However, the problem is not yet solved and these programmes will need to continue for many years to ensure that these children receive an education and grow up in loving homes to become happy and productive citizens.

CHAPTER 11

HIV AND AIDS IN THE WORKPLACE

Ansie Minnaar

KEY CONCEPTS

- morale in the workplace
- AIDS education and prevention programmes
- openness
- non-discrimination
- ethical issues
- patient care
- morbidity and absenteeism, mortality
- staff morale
- benefits
- demand for service

- economic impact
- bill of rights
- workplace response
- UNAIDS
- Code of Good Practice
- the Constitution
- labour legislation
- minimum standards on HIV and AIDS
- consultation
- mainstreaming of HIV and AIDS in the workplace

Taking care of HIV and AIDS patients is emotionally and physically demanding on healthcare workers. The secrecy surrounding the disease, the needs of those living with HIV and AIDS, and the lack of support, all impact on the stress levels of nurses.

(Sengwana 2005)

INTRODUCTION

Globally, an estimated 40 million people are infected with HIV. In less than two years, this figure will leap to 100 million, according to the World Health Organisation (WHO). By 2005, 65 million people will have been infected. Half of the people in this group will be under 25 years old, and will die before they reach the age of 35. Approximately one in every four sexually active person in South Africa is infected. South Africa is believed to be the country with the fastest growing HIV epidemic in the world, with an estimated 2000 new cases every day. It has been said that AIDS is not a disease; it is a development disaster (*Gayle & Gater 2003*). Figure 11.1 shows how HIV and AIDS in the workplace is affecting labour costs globally (*Minnaar 2005*).

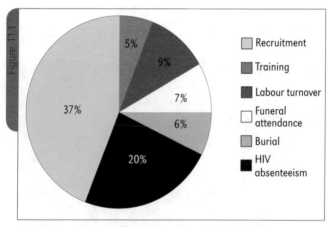

Distribution of increased labour costs due to HIV and AIDS
Source: Freeman 2003:52

The public service must deal with a number of key challenges in order to improve their response to the epidemic. AIDS education and prevention programmes must receive solid, sustained support and become more rigorous and strategic. Active on-going management commitment is needed for a successful response. Partnerships with unions should be actively forged to develop a common vision of how to address the impacts of HIV and AIDS on employees and on service delivery. The adequacy of existing structures should be assessed and the capacity to develop and implement departmental HIV and AIDS programmes should be strengthened and then periodically reviewed. HIV and AIDS policies and programmes should be developed as a matter of urgency in departments that do not have them. Policies should be critically evaluated on a regular basis. Specific issues related to HIV and AIDS should be more explicitly incorporated into the planning and implementation of core departmental functions, as well as into strategies and plans for skills development. Active steps should be taken to encourage the acceptance of employees infected by HIV and AIDS, as well as openness and non-discrimination (*Barrett-Grant et al. 2002*). The next section deals with the projected impact of HIV and AIDS on the health services in the next ten years.

HIV AND AIDS AND THE WORK ENVIRONMENT

Ethical issues and patient care

Nurses may fear treating patients with HIV because they fear infection. Although there are laws to protect people infected with HIV from discrimination, there are still reports of healthcare professionals refusing to care for HIV-positive patients. There are also cases of patients refusing to allow an HIV-infected healthcare professional to care for them, and cases of HIV-positive healthcare workers who have their confidentiality violated, their privileges to practise denied and who lose their jobs. Education on the transmission and prevention of HIV-infection has helped, but the problems still exist.

The risk of HIV transmission to healthcare practitioners from patients is very low, especially if universal precautions are used. However, many healthcare practitioners would like to see all patients tested for HIV so they can better protect themselves. Infection control is discussed in Chapter 5. The risk of HIV transmission from a healthcare practitioner to a patient is even lower than the risk of transmission from an infected patient. However, there have still been proposals for laws that would require all healthcare practitioners to be tested for HIV and to disclose of their status to the public.

Healthcare practitioners cannot allow their personal values and opinions to affect their professional practice. A good understanding of the laws and ethical issues surrounding HIV infection will help healthcare practitioners to make sound ethical judgements and decisions.

Human resources and HIV and AIDS

Public and development sector managers confront endless challenges as they strive to implement their policies. The impact of HIV and AIDS within the workplace will be experienced in many areas, which are detailed in the next section.

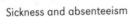

Sickness and absenteeism

As infected employees become ill they will take additional sick leave. This will disrupt the operation of the institution for which they work, which will be amplified when more qualified and experienced employees are infected and absent. Increases in deaths due to HIV and AIDS result in people taking time off work to attend funerals for family members, friends and colleagues. Women employees, due to their socially defined role as caregivers, also have to care for sick children and partners, which may involve time off work.

Death or retirement

The impact on an organisation of the death or retirement of an infected employee has many ramifications. The loss of an employee requires an appropriate replacement to be appointed and trained. For highly qualified staff this is often difficult, particularly in developing economies with skills shortages. Training and recruitment are costly and disrupt operations.

Staff morale

The epidemic may have a negative impact on morale in the workplace. There is a fear of infection and death. There may be resistance to shouldering the additional responsibilities for colleagues who are off sick, away from work or newly recruited and not yet fully functional.

Benefits

Employers and employees will feel the impact of HIV as the cost of employee benefits increases.

Demand for services

The demand for services, particularly for health and welfare services, is likely to increase dramatically. This will have major implications for departments that provide these services, particularly if they already face capacity constraints or are short staffed.

The progression and impact of HIV and AIDS in the workplace

Progression of HIV and AIDS in the workplace	Economic impact of individual case	Economic impact of all cases
Employee becomes infected	No cost to company at this stage (Sick leave days for flu-like illnesses)	No cost to company at this stage
HIV and AIDS-related morbidity begins	• Sick leave and absenteeism increases • Work performance declines due to employee illness • Overtime and contractor's wages increase to compensate for absenteeism • Use of company's onsite health clinic increases • Payouts from medical aid schemes increase • Employee requires attention of human resources and employee assistance personnel (EAP)	• Overall productivity declines • Overall labour costs increase • Medical aid premiums increase (high demands) • Additional medical staff need to be employed (health clinics on site) • Managers begin to spend time and resources on HIV and AIDS-related issues • HIV and AIDS interventions are designed and implemented • Restructuring jobs and reorganising workstations • Adjusting working hours and leave • Providing specialised supervision, training and support
Employee leaves workforce due to death, medical boarding or voluntary resignation	• Payout from death benefit or life insurance scheme is claimed • Pension benefits are claimed • Absenteeism due to funerals and support to HIV and AIDS affected • Funeral expenses	

Table 11.1

Progression of HIV and AIDS in the workplace	Economic impact of individual case	Economic impact of all cases
	• Company loans to employees not paid back • Demoralised workers affected by HIV and AIDS	• Payouts from pension fund cause increases in contributions • Returns on investments are reduced (e.g. training) • Morale, stress and discipline are disrupted by deaths in companies
Company recruits a replacement employee	• Recruitment costs • Vacant positions • Cost of overtime	• Additional staff are brought in • Wages increase as a response to market demands
Company trains the new employee	• Pre-employment training • In-service training to bring new employees up to standard	• Additional training staff and resources needed
New employee joins the workforce	• Performance is low while new employee comes up to speed • On the job training	• Reduction in experience, skill and performance of the workforce • Production, productivity is disrupted

Source: Freeman 2003: Toolkit: Managing HIV & AIDS in the workplace

THE GOVERNING FRAMEWORK FOR A RESPONSE TO HIV AND AIDS

One clause of the Bill of Rights contained within the Constitution protects the rights of every person to equality, dignity, privacy and fair labour practices. In the context of HIV and AIDS the right to equality is critical, since infected people are often stigmatised and discriminated against. Section 9(1) seeks to ensure equal treatment of all persons, including those living with HIV and AIDS. Furthermore, sections 9(3) and 9(4) offer protection against unfair discrimination to people with HIV and AIDS. Therefore, nurses may not discriminate against HIV and AIDS patients when providing nursing care (*Mubangizi 2004*).

Any workplace response to HIV and AIDS must therefore be based on an understanding of the rights of the infected person. This requires knowledge of:

- international guidelines for responding to HIV and AIDS
- the South African legislative and policy framework
- public service legislation and policy on HIV and AIDS.

International guidelines

There are a number of important international guidelines that have been developed to guide the response of governments to HIV and AIDS. These are the most significant.

The UNAIDS HIV and AIDS and Human Rights International Guidelines (1998)

These are international guidelines to assist states in creating a positive, rights-based response to HIV and AIDS, which is effective in reducing the transmission of HIV, reducing the impact of the epidemic and which is consistent with human rights and fundamental freedoms.

The SADC Code of Good Practice on HIV and AIDS and Employment (1997)

The SADC Code was developed through a consultative tripartite process and adopted at a meeting of ministers of labour in Pretoria, South Africa in August 1997. Although the Code is not a legally binding document, all those who were signatories to it agreed that:

- The national and regional implications of the HIV and AIDS epidemic meant that there was a need to have regional employment standards.
- All member countries should develop tripartite national codes that are reflected in national law.

The International Labour Organisation (ILO) Code of Practice on HIV and AIDS and the World of Work (2001)

This Code binds all employers and employees in the private and public sectors and all aspects of work, formal and informal. The following standards can be used in developing a response to HIV and AIDS in the workplace:

- HIV and AIDS must be recognised as a workplace issue.
- Responses to HIV and AIDS must be based on the principle of non-discrimination.

- Gender equality must be pursued as part of any HIV and AIDS response.
- Every employee has a right to a healthy and safe working environment.
- Social dialogue between employers, workers, their representatives, government and people living with HIV and AIDS must take place on HIV and AIDS issues.
- There must be no HIV screening of job applicants or employees.
- Every employee has the right to confidentiality regarding their HIV status.
- Workers must be enabled to continue working for as long as possible.
- Workplaces must promote HIV prevention.
- Care and support should be provided to infected workers (*Barrett-Grant et al. 2002*).

South African laws

South Africa has a good legislative framework for responding to HIV and AIDS in the workplace. Some of the most important pieces of legislation are described below, including how the principles established within international law have been integrated into South African domestic law and policies.

The Constitution

The South African Constitution Act, No. 108 of 1996 is the overiding law of the country and all other laws must comply with it. The Bill of Rights within the Constitution sets out a number of specific provisions that protect workplace rights. Section 23(1) states that 'Everyone has the right to fair labour practices'. There are also more general rights, which apply to the employment relationship, such as the right to equality and non-discrimination (section 9), and privacy (section 13).

Labour legislation

There are a number of important labour statutes, though only one of them, the Employment Equity Act, specifically refers to HIV and AIDS. However, all are general enough to cover most HIV and AIDS-related problems that may arise in the workplace. These Acts apply to all employees, except those employed by the South African National Defence Force (SANDF), the National Intelligence Agency and the Secret Service. The relevant labour statutes are covered below.

The Employment Equity Act, No. 55 of 1998

This Act aims at ensuring equality and non-discrimination in the workplace through anti-discrimination measures and affirmative action provisions. It also has two clauses that expressly refer to HIV and AIDS:

- a prohibition on unfair discrimination based on 'HIV status'
- a prohibition on HIV testing without Labour Court authorisation.

The Labour Relations Act, No. 66 of 1995

This Act is aimed at regulating the relationships between employees, trade unions and employers, for example, by setting out when trade unions may meet with their members at the workplace. It also regulates the resolution of disputes between employers and employees and sets out the rights of workers with regard to dismissal.

The Occupational Health and Safety Act, No. 85 of 1993

This Act places a duty on all employers to ensure that, as far as is reasonably practicable, the working environment is safe and healthy for employees. For example, employers are required to provide safety equipment such as latex gloves to prevent the transmission of HIV during an accident involving a blood spill in the workplace.

The Compensation for Occupational Injuries and Diseases Act, No. 130 of 1993

This Act gives every employee the right to apply for compensation if injured in the course and scope of their employment. This would include compensation for HIV infection if it can be shown that the employee was infected in the course and scope of their employment.

Other relevant legislation

There are also a number of other pieces of legislation, which, although not directly employment related, have an impact on the management of HIV and AIDS in the workplace.

The Promotion of Equality and Prevention of Unfair Discrimination Act, No. 4 of 2000

This Act sets out measures for dealing with various forms of unfair discrimination and inequality. It also sets out the steps that must be taken to promote equality. This Act is broad enough to cover unfair discrimination based on HIV status. It applies to all agencies, including those not covered by existing labour legislation, namely the SANDF, the Secret Service and the National Intelligence Agency, providing protection against discrimination against employees living with HIV and AIDS.

The Medical Schemes Act, No. 131 of 1998

This Act is regulated by Government Gazette 20556, 20 October 1999, medical schemes. It states that a medical scheme may not unfairly discriminate, directly or indirectly, against any person on the basis of their HIV status. This Act also allows the Minister of Health to gazette a minimum standard of benefits to be provided to members of the medical scheme.

There are a number of policies that define good practice related to factors that have implications for HIV and AIDS.

The Code of Good Practice on Key Aspects of HIV and AIDS and Employment

This is attached to both the Labour Relations and Employment Equity Acts. It is essentially a standard setting out the content and scope of an appropriate response to HIV and AIDS in the workplace.

The Code has two objectives:

- to set out guidelines for employers and trade unions to implement to ensure that individuals infected with HIV are not unfairly discriminated against in the workplace
- to provide guidelines for employers, employees and trade unions on how to manage HIV and AIDS within the workplace.

The Code of Good Practice on Dismissal, which is a code attached to the Labour Relations Act, provides guidelines on, for example, when and how an employer may dismiss an employee for incapacity.

The Draft Code of Good Practice on Key Aspects of Disability and Employment is currently being finalised by the Department of Labour. This code will give detailed guidelines on how to accommodate disabled employees, such as those with advanced HIV disease and how to adapt their working environments.

Rights established by the legal and policy framework

A number of the rights within international law are also protected in South African laws and policies. The rights of employees living with HIV and AIDS include the right to:

- equality and non-discrimination, which includes protection on the basis of 'HIV status' (ref. the Constitution, the Employment Equity Act and the Promotion of Equality and the Prevention of Unfair Discrimination Act)
- be tested only following Labour Court authorisation (ref. the Employment Equity Act)
- privacy and confidentiality (ref. the Constitution and common law)
- a safe working environment and compensation if injured at work (ref. the Occupational Health and Safety Act and the Compensation for Occupational Injuries and Diseases Act)
- equal access to employee benefits (ref. the Medical Schemes Act)
- a minimum level of medical aid benefits from their medical aid scheme (ref. the Medical Schemes Act)
- be protected from unfair dismissal based on HIV status (ref. the Labour Relations Act) (*Barrett-Grant et al. 2002*).

The Public Service Regulations, 2001 incorporated new Minimum Standards on HIV and AIDS.

Table 11.2

- That the working environment takes account of the personal circumstances of employees living with HIV and AIDS;
- That steps are taken to identify and reduce the risk of HIV transmission in the working environment;
- That steps are taken to manage occupational exposure to HIV and AIDS;
- That measures are taken to prohibit unfair discrimination and promote non-discrimination on the basis of HIV status or AIDS;
- That HIV testing of a public servant is prohibited;
- That voluntary counselling and testing for HIV (VCT) is encouraged;
- That the confidentiality of HIV status is maintained;
- That health promotion programmes are introduced to deal with HIV and AIDS prevention, and care and acceptance of people living with HIV and AIDS;
- That support for HIV and AIDS policies and programmes is established through allocating responsibilities, human and financial resources, structures and communication strategies; and
- That measures are put into place to monitor and evaluate HIV & AIDS policies and programmes

Source: Barrett-Grant et al. 2002

DISTINCTION BETWEEN POLICIES, PROGRAMMES AND PROJECTS

There is often confusion about the differences between a policy, a programme, and a project. A policy in its most general definition is a set of guidelines to meet certain goals. A programme is a structured process of attempting to meet those goals. Programmes consist of a portfolio of projects. A project is a more specific way of meeting the goals of the programme and ultimately the goals of the policy.

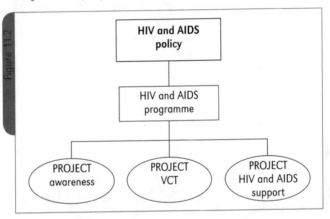

A model illustrating the interrelationship between a policy, a programme and a project

Developing an HIV and AIDS policy: the eight key stages

1 Consultation between employers, staff and unions
2 Establishment of a committee on HIV and AIDS
3 Committee gets expert advice on HIV and AIDS
4 Policy draft: policy content should aim at:
   • non-discrimination
   • HIV testing, confidentiality and disclosure
   • a safe working environment
   • compensation
   • benefits
   • grievance procedures
   • management of HIV and AIDS in the workplace

w where she got the HIV virus from. Was it from the work-
operating theatre? Or somewhere else? She gave it some
some time, but with no clear answer emerging, she stopped
this. Now X just lives from day to day and the child is doing
ol with reasonable health. X is paying special attention to
n and is not on antiretrovirals. She is looking after herself,
th a circle of friends supporting her. She picked up her life and
g every single day.

disturbing fact is that X realised that if she had stayed at the
she would be dead by now because she was treated in such an
way. That is not the way to treat our own. The nursing staff and
anagers should not judge HIV-positive nurses. All nurses should
k and reflect on how care was given to nurse colleagues in the
ce, particularly those who are sick and who are struggling with
AIDS. Nurses affected and infected with HIV and AIDS should
ured and cared for by their colleagues.

5 Consultation on draft policy between employers, employees and trade unions

6 Final policy developed

7 Policy implementation (consultation and identification on the different projects)

8 Ongoing evaluation, consultation and improvement of HIV and AIDS policy.

STRATEGIES FOR IMPLEMENTATION OF PROGRAMMES AND MAINSTREAMING HIV AND AIDS IN THE WORKPLACE

Further research needs to be done on the effect of HIV and AIDS on health delivery systems, in order to establish the requirements for support, guidance, counselling and care to dying nurses. This information is critical to nurse managers. Nurse managers need to know how well and for how long HIV-infected nurses will be able to work, so that they can plan service delivery. There should be sufficient additional support and guidance given to nursing managers, and additional nurses should be provided to cope with the demands of HIV and AIDS-positive nurses

A strategy for mainstreaming HIV and AIDS in the nursing workplace needs to be urgently developed and taken up by nurse managers and trainers. There are three components to this strategy. Firstly, nurse managers must demonstrate leadership in handling HIV and AIDS issues, and provide care for nurses affected by HIV and AIDS. Secondly, health services must lead other stakeholders in responding to HIV and AIDS. Finally, on a personal level, managers must provide role models by not discriminating against people who are living with AIDS.

Nurse managers should raise HIV and AIDS awareness at trade union meetings and ensure that trade unions place HIV and AIDS leadership on the bargaining agenda. Management should be requested to establish HIV and AIDS structures and clearly delegate responsibility for these structures. A permanent HIV and AIDS slot is needed in staff meeting agendas to allow all staff access to progress reports. Ensure that the HIV and AIDS Committee has the opportunity to report on progress and to table their plans at the annual planning meetings.

Nurse managers need specialised skills for dealing with the impact of HIV and AIDS on nurses and health services. This training needs to take high priority. Awareness programmes should be a priority for nurse managers, as well as for those in all the public services in South Africa. It is estimated that by 2010, 15% of highly skilled employees will have contracted HIV and

AIDS. This will have a major impact on staff morale and on skills levels in the health service.

Nurses are increasingly involved with HIV and AIDS patient care. Workplace issues also change when new diseases emerge. Nurse managers and nurses need to be aware of these changes and must be able to respond to and to deal with issues that face nurses in the workplace. Nurses have regular and prolonged contact with HIV and AIDS patients and must provide extensive physical care and emotional support to many patients dying of AIDS. It is clear that nurses are experiencing occupational stress, fatigue and symptoms of occupational burnout. This may be exacerbated by the fear of HIV transmission from accidental exposure to infected body fluids.

Furthermore, stress may be associated with deficiencies in AIDS-specific training and knowledge. Nurses might see themselves as incompetent to render nursing care to these patients. Studies have shown that nurses express negative perceptions and experiences regarding HIV and AIDS nursing. Nurses feel helpless or powerlessness when they care for HIV and AIDS patients. However, they also feel empathy and compassion towards these patients, along with pity and melancholy.

More proactive initiatives are needed to help nurses cope with the burden of HIV and AIDS nursing care. Healthcare organisations should provide stress management courses, nurses support groups and recognition for nurse's work. In order for nurses' to give quality nursing care, hospitals and other health services organisations must provide a working environment where sufficient knowledge transfer and enough supplies are provided to enable nurses to do their work – to care for patients.

CONCLUSION

There are large financial benefits and gains for companies and other sectors who keep their workforce healthy for as long as possible. This reduces the time managers and human resource personnel spend coping with employee deaths and high staff turnover, and also reduces the impact on staff morale and motivation. Keeping the workforce healthy creates more time for management to implement strategies to cope with the epidemic, such as training replacement employees, shifting to less labour-intensive technologies and managing the loss of overall workforce skill and experiences caused by HIV and AIDS (*Rosen et al. 2000*).

The following case study may act as a guide for managers.

A CASE STUDY

X'S WORKING LIFE

X is a nurse who had worked in a c of a public hospital. The tea room w day X announced her pregnancy and now aged seven. However, the baby At 18 months the baby was tested fo X was shattered. Where did the baby found that she was also HIV-positive. 'V

X told her husband that she was HIV-po with three kids to care for. She turned to th This was a very difficult time for X. She s was happening to her.

While she was grappling with these huge is back to her work as a nurse auxiliary at the l her enemies. They rejected her. They were gos not speak to anyone. But she had to speak to nurse manager about her HIV status. Unfortu The next time she reported for duty, everythin leagues looked at her in a different way. Most c avoided her, as if they were afraid that she woul

There were supportive people in the workplace. S special and they could be described with words s supportive and very kind.

However, back in the operating theatre, it was qu Her colleagues did not understand. When her child couldn't come to work, she was crucified, and they c they gossiped. Everyone would know, at her return, t ill again. Her previous friends and colleagues were kil mistrust and the ongoing gossiping.

She realised that she had to leave the workplace or she So she resigned from her job, her only income since her hu them. This was hard. X was now faced with the realities of and providing for three children and herself. 'God, what n She found consolation in another church group who accep was part of a group again.

X did not kn place, in th thought for dwelling on fine at sch her nutriti together w she is livin

The most hospital, uncaring nurse m look ba workpla HIV an be nur

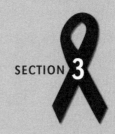

SECTION 3

CHAPTER 12

HIV AND AIDS PATIENTS AND CRITICAL CARE NURSING

Ansie Minnaar

> As more patients are receiving antiretroviral regimens,
> the intensive care nurse can expect to see
> more complications of this therapy.
>
> *(Morris et al. 2006)*

INTRODUCTION

Respiratory failure due to PCP (pneumocystis pneumonia) used to be the most common disorder for which AIDS patients were admitted to ICU, often with a fatal outcome. However, the outlook of HIV-infected patients has improved in most countries with improved access to antiretrovirals. In the past ten years our perception of HIV and AIDS has changed from seeing the infection as an invariably fatal disease to seeing it as a manageable chronic illness (*Rosen 2005*). In the early days of HIV the prognosis for survival was poor, and patients often declined ICU care. However, during the early 1990s, survival increased after mechanical ventilation was offered. Treatment of HIV and AIDS patients in ICU continued to evolve. The incidence of PCP declined as a result of prophylaxis with bactrim and the use of corticosteroids for respiratory failure in pneumocystis pneumonia, and fewer patients were admitted to ICU. With the introduction of combination antiretroviral therapy, the incidence pf PCP and other opportunistic infections declined still further.

It is now clear that when most HIV-infected patients who use antiretroviral therapy die, they are increasingly likely to die of non-AIDS-associated disorders, such as end-stage liver disease if they are co-infected with hepatitis B or C (*Rosen 2005*). This will change the pattern of ICU admissions for HIV patients. Antiretroviral therapy itself can be toxic and some drug reactions may require ICU admission. There may also be complex drug interactions in the ICU in patients on antiretrovirals. Importantly, the immune reconstruction that follows the start of antiretroviral therapy may cause an accelerated inflammatory response to active infections (*Rosen 2005*).

The overall management and prognosis of patients infected with HIV has changed dramatically over the course of the AIDS epidemic as a result of antiretroviral therapy and prophylaxis against opportunistic infections.

HUMAN IMMUNODEFICIENCY VIRUS INFECTION

To be diagnosed with AIDS, a person with HIV infection must have one of the indicator conditions discussed in Table 2.1 on page 30 (Stage 4). The rate of progression from HIV-positive status to AIDS is significantly higher in people who are not receiving antiretroviral therapy. The higher the CD4 count and the lower the viral load, the lower the risk of progression to AIDS (*Morton et al. 2005*).

REASONS FOR HIV AND AIDS PATIENTS TO BE ADMITTED TO ICU

The most common reason for ICU admission is respiratory failure. Other reasons might be diseases such as central nervous system dysfunction, sepsis, bleeding, drug overdose, cardiopulmonary arrest, renal failure, pancreatitis, lactic acidosis, hypersensitivity syndrome, diabetic ketoacidosis, post operation, trauma, hypertensive emergency, angina, cardiac dysrhythmia, and thrombotic thrombocytopenic purpura.

ANTIRETROVIRAL THERAPY

The availability of treatment with antiretrovirals has affected the presentation and outcome of critical care patients infected with HIV and suffering from AIDS. Patients on antiretrovirals who are admitted to ICUs characteristically present with different syndromes from patients who are not receiving these drugs. Drug toxicity, drug interaction and immune reconstitution inflammatory syndrome (IRIS) are associated with antiretroviral therapy. It is extremely important that ICU nurses recognise and understand the implications of these illnesses and have a clear understanding of them in order to offer optimal care and accurate diagnosis of patients.

EPIDEMIOLOGY OF HIV-INFECTED PATIENTS IN THE ICU

Changes are reflected in mortality and ICU admission rates, changes in predictors of ICU mortality, changes in ICU diagnosis and lastly changes in patient characteristics.

There have been major changes in the mortality rates and ICU admission rates of HIV-infected patients over the years, which have been influenced by various factors such as patient him/herself, and the health service's attitude towards care and service delivery. There is little information on this that is specific to South Africa, so information will be taken from USA sources (*Morris et al. 2006*) and will deal with HIV and AIDS from 1981 to the time of writing.

Between 1981 and 1985, the majority of HIV-infected patients admitted to ICU had pneumocystis pneumonia (PCP). The mortality was high and those who were discharged, survived for an average of only seven months. During 1984 the admission rates to ICUs dropped, possibly because both doctors and patients saw ICU care as futile and withdrew critical care. However, the introduction of corticosteroids in the treatment of PCP resulted in a significant fall in mortality rates of those infected with HIV.

Between 1986 and 1988, mortality rates increased again, and between 1989 and 1991 there was an increase in ICU admission rates. Hereafter ICU admission rates remained stable, and between 1992 and 1995 the mortality rate improved again. Between 1996 and now, mortality and admission rates have changed again in the USA. Both mortality and ICU admissions have decreased. This is probably because increasing numbers of peope are taking antiretrovirals, so ICU admissions are no longer for AIDS-related illness.

There have also been changes in predictors of ICU mortality. Factors predicting mortality include the need for mechanical ventilation or a diagnosis of PCP, while a non-AIDS-associated diagnosis, a serum albumin level more than 2.6 g/dl in liver disease, and an Acute Physiology and Chronic Health Evaluation II score of more than 13 (APACHE II) are associated with an increase in survival to discharge (*Morris et al. 2006*). The APACHE II score is used to assess severity of illness on admission. The score uses physiological parameters such as body temperature, serum electrolyte levels and level of consciousness and allocates weights to the different parameters. The APACHE II predicts mortality with approximately 85% accuracy and low scores are associated with improved survival (*Gardner & Sibthorpe 2002*).

Factors such as mechanical ventilation, low serum albumin, and PCP predicted an increased mortality rate before the introduction of combination antiretrovirals (*Morris et al. 2006*).

Bacterial pneumonia and bacterial sepsis are now becoming more common admission diagnoses in ICU, as is end-stage liver disease. Pulmonary hypertension and lung cancer and complications of chemotherapy are also more common reasons for admission, since these conditions seem to have increased with the introduction of combination antiretrovirals.

The in-hospital mortality of patients with pneumocystis pneumonia who required mechanical ventilation in ICU is the highest, followed by neurological disorders. Sepsis is a very common cause of death among HIV-positive patients and is the third most common reason for admission to ICU. Septic shock and multiple organ failure are common among HIV patients admitted to ICU (*Bhagwanjee et al. 1997*).

In the USA at least, HIV status is no longer a consideration when a patient is being assessed for admission to ICU.

CLINICAL ILLNESS OF THE HIV AND AIDS PATIENT IN ICU

There is a strong relationship between CD4 count and clinical illness, shown in Table 12.1. The primary goal of management in critical ill HIV and AIDS patients is the prevention or resolution of opportunistic infections and nosocomial infections. Opportunistic infections are the leading cause of death in patients with HIV and AIDS, and therefore, prevention is the cornerstone of treatment in ICU. Treatment is aimed at support of the involved system or systems. The current organisms for which prophylaxis is strongly recommended include *P. jiroveci*, *Mycobacterium tuberculosis*, and *Toxoplasma gondii*.

The intensive care nurse should be on the alert for the following problems when nursing HIV and AIDS patients:

- the high risk of infections related to HIV immunodeficiency
- the risk of impaired gas exchange related to alveolar-capillary membrane changes in *Pneumocystis jiroveci* pneumonia
- the risk of dehydration and fluid volume deficiency related to diarrhoea and dysphagia
- the risk of infection transmission

- patient anxiety related to critical illness and fear of death
- any deficiency in knowledge related to HIV and AIDS
- the risk of disturbed thought processes due to infection of the central nervous system (*Morton et al. 2005*).

The relationship between CD4 count and HIV and AIDS complications

Table 12.1	CD4 count	Infectious complications	Non-infectious complications
	>500	Acute retroviral syndrome Candidal vaginitis	Persistent generalised lymphadenopathy Guillian-Barré syndrome Myopathy Aseptic meningitis
	200–500	Pneumoccocal and other bacterial pneumonia Pulmonary tuberculosis (TB) (this can occur at any CD4 count in South Africa)	Cervical intraepithelial neoplasia Cervical cancer
		Herpes zoster	B-cell lymphoma
		Oropharyngeal candidiasis (thrush)	Anaemia
		Crytosporidiosis self-limited	Mononeuronal multiplex
		Kaposi's sarcoma	Idiopathic thrombocytopenic purpura
		Oral hairy leukoplakia	Hodgkin's lymphoma Lymphocytic interstitial pneumonitis
	<200	*Pneumocystis jiroveci* pneumonia	Wasting
		Disseminated histoplasmosis and coccidioidomycosis	Peripheral neuropathy
		Miliary/extrapulmonary TB	HIV-associated dementia

CD4 count	Infectious complications	Non-infectious complications
	Progressive multifocal leukoencephalopathy	Cardiomypathy Vacuolar myelopathy Progressive polyradiculopathy
<100	Disseminated herpes simplex Toxoplasmosis Cryptococcosis Cryptosporidiosis, chronic Microsporidiosis Candidal oesophagitis	
<50	Disseminated cytomegalovirus Disseminated Mycrobacterium avium complex	Central nervous system lymphoma

Source: Morton, et al. 2005

Respiratory system

PCP usually occurs when the CD4 count is less than 200 cells/μl. It presents as a respiratory illness with breathlessness, night sweats and weight loss. Complications may include respiratory failure, pneumothorax and chronic pulmonary disease. Chest X-ray shows bilateral shadowing and lung function tests show reduced lung volumes with decreased compliance and diminished diffusion capacity. Oxygen saturation measurements can be more helpful than lung function tests. If PCP is suspected, fibreoptic bronchoscopy should be performed. First-line treatment is with co-trimoxazole, oral or intravenous. Corticosteroids should always be used. Second-line therapy is pentamidine. Respiratory support and supplementary oxygen are invariably required. Continuous positive airway pressure (CPAP) and positive end-expiratory pressure (PEEP) might be needed. PEEP can cause pneumothorax.

Cavitatory lung disease can be due to pyogenic bacterial lung abscess, pulmonary tuberculosis (TB), fungal infections and Nocardia species. Kaposi's sarcoma and lymphoma can also affect the lung. Adenophathy can lead to tracheobronchial obstruction or compression of the great vessels.

HIV directly affects the lungs, causing a destructive pulmonary syndrome similar to emphysema (*Avidan et al. 2000*).

Central nervous system (CNS)

The neurological diseases in AIDS range from AIDS dementia to infectious and neoplastic involvement. Three cerebral diseases complicate AIDS, namely cerebral toxoplasmosis, primary CNS lymphoma and progressive multifocal leucoencephalopathy. Any focal lesion may increase intracerebral pressure. The spinal cord may be involved, with peripheral neuropathy and myopathy with cytomegalovirus or HIV infection itself. Cryptococcus neoformans, HIV and TB can all cause meningitis (*Avidan et al. 2000*).

Other important clinical illnesses

Cardiac involvement in the development of HIV disease is common. Up to 50% of HIV and AIDS patients have abnormal echocardiographic findings and about 25% present with pericardial effusion. Myocarditis is common and could be caused by toxoplasmosis, cryptococcus, coxackie virus, cytomegalovirus, lymphoma, aspergillus and HIV itself (*Avidan et al 2000*).

HIV AND AIDS AND PAIN

Pain is an important problem in HIV and AIDS patients. Pain can occur at any stage but is most important in the advanced stages of the disease. The type of pain associated with HIV and AIDS is headache, herpes simplex virus infection, back pain, post-herpetic neuralgia, throat pain and abdominal pain. Painful peripheral neuropathy is the most common neurological disorder associated with HIV and AIDS (*Avidan et al. 2000*).

To treat this the pain needs to be localised and characterised. Causes, such as infections and malignancies, should be ruled out. The psychological and emotional contribution to pain should also be considered. Assess pain by history taking, physical examination, medication identification, and history of substance use or misuse, and neurological and psychological assessment. Current pain management includes non-narcotic analgesics, narcotic analgesics, tricyclic antidepressants, anticonvulsants, physical therapy and psychological treatment. Treat pain using the same principles as cancer-related pain treatment (*Avidan et al. 2000*).

ICU ADMISSION FOR ANTIRETROVIRAL-RELATED TOXICITIES

With the introduction of antiretrovirals in South Africa, ICU nurses can expect to see more complications of this therapy. These drugs cause a number of side effects and syndromes, some of which can be fatal. The main problems that may result in ICU admission in those using antiretroviral are lactic acidosis, hypersensitivity syndrome, drug toxicities and atherosclerosis and cardiovascular disease.

Lactic acidosis was first described in the 1990s and can occur with any of the nucleotide reverse transcriptase inhibitors (NRTIs) but is most often associated with stavudine d4T. Lactic acidosis results from mitochondrial toxicity caused by these agents and is believed to be secondary to impaired synthesis of adenosine triphosphate-generating mitochondrial enzymes. The mortality rate is high, at 77%. Risk factors for the development of lactic acidosis are: a creatinine clearance of less than 70 ml/min and a CD4 cell count of less than 250 cells/µl. Abdominal pain, dyspnoea, nausea, and vomiting are common symptoms. Furthermore, patients also may present with myalgias or peripheral neuropathies, hepatic steatosis and an elevation of transaminases. Some patients progress to life-threatening organ failure, including respiratory failure and haemodynamic instability.

The serum lactate should be tested in any patient presenting with symptoms of lactic acidosis. The accuracy of the test depends on the blood collection technique. Blood should be taken without a tourniquet into a pre-chilled fluoride-oxalate tube and transported immediately to the laboratory. Improper collection techniques can result in false elevated lactate levels. An initial lactate level of more than 9 mmol/l is associated with a high risk of death. Bicarbonate therapy and haemodialysis may be necessary.

Hypersensitivity syndrome is caused by several antiretroviral agents. Patients typically present with fever, rash, nausea, and vomiting and abdominal pain. They can become hypotensive and develop acute interstitial pneumonitis and respiratory failure. Antiretroviral therapy should be discontinued immediately. Nevirapine can cause hypersensitivity syndrome and in severe cases, patients develop fulminant hepatitis and hepatic necrosis or severe skin involvement, including Stevens-Johnson syndrome and toxic epidermal necrolysis (*Morlat in Morris et al. 2006*).

Protease inhibitors may cause hepatitis and pancreatitis, which could result in admission to ICU.

Immune reconstitution inflammatory syndrome (IRIS) can sometimes be life-threatening. It may be difficult to distinguish between this syndrome and acute opportunistic infections. Patients experience paradoxical worsening of infections after starting antiretrovirals. For example, in a patient with isolated pulmonary TB, starting antiretrovirals may trigger meningitis, pericarditis or lymphadenitis. Both PCP and cytomegalovirus infection may flare up in patients receiving secondary prophylaxis.

As antiretroviral use and so life expectancy increases, there will be HIV patients who have cardiovascular problems that require ICU admission. Patients on protease inhibitors also develop lipodystrophy as a side effect of these drugs, which could cause cardiovascular disease.

Using antiretrovirals in the ICU

Administration of antiretrovirals in the intensive care unit is complex and potentially dangerous but may be associated with benefits in survival that could justify its use (*Morlat in Morris et al. 2006*).

When an HIV patient on antiretrovirals is admitted to ICU, a decision needs to be made about whether or not to continue the treatment. However, a patient admitted to ICU may not be aware of their HIV status and may be diagnosed during this admission. The question now is whether or not to start antiretrovirals in a situation where there is limited availability of intravenous medication, erratic gastric absorption, potential HIV resistance, possible non-compliance after discharge and multiple drug interaction, side effects and overlapping toxicities.

HIV TRANSMISSION TO HEALTHCARE STAFF IN THE ICU'S

The risk of HIV transmission to healthcare workers is low if standard precautions and transmission-based precautions are followed.

Standard precautions to be taken in ICU

- Wash hands after touching blood, body fluids, secretions, excretions, and contaminated items, regardless of wearing gloves. Wash hands immediately after gloves are removed, between patient contacts, and whenever indicated to prevent transfer of microorganisms to other patients. Use plain soap for routine hand washing and an antimicrobial agent for specific circumstances.
- Wear clean, nonsterile gloves when touching blood, body fluids, excretions or secretions, contaminated items, mucous membranes, and non-intact skin. Change gloves between patients and between tasks.
- Wear a mask, eye protection or a face shield during procedures and care activities that are likely to generate splashes or sprays or blood or body fluids. Use a gown to protect skin and prevent soiling of clothes.
- Ensure that patient care equipment that is soiled with blood or body fluids, secretions and excretions is handled carefully to prevent transfer of microorganisms. Clean appropriately.

- Use adequate environmental controls to ensure that routine care, cleaning and disinfection procedures are followed.
- Handle the transportation and processing of linen soiled with blood and body fluids, excretions and secretions in a manner that prevents exposure and contamination of clothing and transfer of organisms.
- Use preventative measures when using needles, sharps and scalpels and place them in appropriate containers.

Airborne precautions

- Place the patient in a private room with negative air pressure.
- Use respiratory protection when entering the room of patients with known or suspected tuberculosis.
- Transport the patient out of the room only when necessary and place a surgical mask on the patient if possible.
- Consult infection control for preventative strategies.

Droplet precautions

- Use a private room, if available. Wear a mask when working within a metre of the patient
- Transport the patient out of the room only when necessary and place a surgical mask on the patient if possible.

Contact precautions

- Use a private room, if available. Wear a mask when working within a metre of the patient
- Transport the patient out of the room only when necessary and place a surgical mask on the patient if possible.
- Wear a gown if contact with infectious agent is likely or patient has diarrhoea, an ileostomy, colostomy or wound drainage not contained by a dressing (*Morton et al. 2005*).

CONCLUSION

We are now entering the third decade of HIV with still no cure in sight. Rigorous infection control practices are imperative in situations where nurses and doctors are in contact with potentially seropositive patients.

The introduction of effective antiretroviral therapy means that HIV patients are living longer, but also that they may experience drug reactions that require ICU admission. These patients may also develop conditions that are not related to HIV, such as end-stage liver disease if co-infected with hepatitis B or C, or cardiac disease, that require ICU admission. Decisions around ICU admission are no longer based on a patient's HIV status.

CHAPTER 13

HOME-BASED NURSING CARE

Ansie Minnaar

KEY CONCEPTS

- home and community care
- palliative care
- counselling
- VCT
- spiritual support
- activities of daily living
- community volunteers
- home-based healthcare workers

> HIV and AIDS have burrowed deeper into the social
> and economic fault lines of communities and societies,
> and it is widening those fissures further.
>
> *(UNAIDS 2002)*

INTRODUCTION

Most people with HIV and AIDS in South Africa are poor and therefore do not have easy access to antiretrovirals and so eventually need palliative care. Economic constraints mean that home-based care is one of the best approaches to HIV and AIDS care in South Africa. However, this should not be regarded as a cheap solution. Home-based care in South Africa at the moment is not provided by government, but the concept is supported. This form of care is generally provided by non-governmental organisations (NGOs) who work with people in the community. Caregivers are usually paid, but care is also provided by unpaid people with a strong sense of community responsibility. Home-based carers often receive training through

NGOs. However, they many not dispense medication, so need to work closely with local clinics and doctors.

HOME AND COMMUNITY CARE

Home-based care is an essential part of our response to the HIV and AIDS epidemic. The Department of Health guidelines stipulate that the home-based care approach should be one of integrated home and community-based care services (*DOH 2001*). Figure 13.1 outlines the integrated approach.

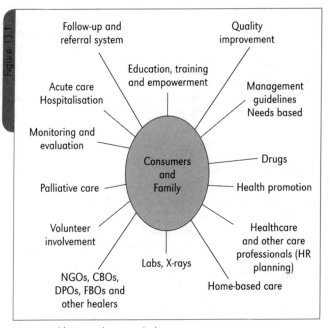

Integrated home and community-base

Source: Adapted from Department of Health (2001:27)

HOME-BASED CARE OF HIV AND AIDS PATIENTS IN THE COMMUNITY

Home-based care can relieve the burden on an already stretched healthcare system. Hospital bed occupancy has increased by over 55% since the HIV epidemic started. Care at home can be provided by family carers, trained volunteers, or health and social workers. There are benefits for the patient because they are nursed in a familiar environment.

The specific objectives of home-based care are:

- to strengthen HIV prevention
- to establish greater involvement of family and community members in the care of HIV and AIDS patients
- to reduce the impact of HIV on TB and HIV-related diseases and nosocomial infections
- to improve the level of HIV and AIDS care to vulnerable and poor people.

Currently, many of the home-based organisations are faith-based and therefore also provide the patient with spiritual care. Both medical and spiritual factors are important in HIV and AIDS care.

Programme interventions should include:

- medical and palliative care of opportunistic infections, treatment of sexually transmitted infections and prophylactic treatment and nursing care
- counselling on VCT, advice on living positively with HIV and AIDS, prevention of HIV transmission through safe sex, and discussion of treatment options
- HIV counselling and testing (VCT) and HIV and AIDS awareness programmes in order to motivate for behavioural change as a prevention strategy
- social, material and spiritual support by specialised organisations, particularly support for mothers and children (*Campbell 2004*).

Assessment of the patient should include:

- the ability to carry out activities of daily living (ADL) such as:
  - distance walked without discomfort
  - ability to get in and out of bed without difficulty
  - ability to get dressed and undressed alone
  - ability to wash without help
  - ability to feed him/herself, including preparing food
  - ability to use the toilet on his/her own
- control over the bladder and bowels
- sight and hearing.

Community volunteers and workers who have had training as AIDS counsellors and in home-based care can provide counselling for HIV and

AIDS patients, follow up for patients on TB treatment, and education on HIV and AIDS for patients and relatives. They can also identify and support orphan-headed households, and identify vulnerable households. They are able to refer patients for further medical treatment where necessary.

CARING FOR HIV AND AIDS IN CHILDREN

Confirm that the child is HIV positive before offering home-based care. A care worker who is trained in the management of opportunistic infections should then visit the child every month. Counselling and health education should be provided for the parents and the child. The child should be provided with one month's supply of prophylactic co-trimoxazole and multivitamins. Opportunistic infections are diagnosed and treated according to Department of Health guidelines. Where necessary, provide antipyretic medication and oral rehydration.

The most common illnesses in HIV-positive children are:

- chronic cough
- dermatitis
- recurrent or prolonged fever
- lymphadenopathy
- recurrent diarrhoea
- oral candidiasis
- pneumonia
- otitis media
- candidial oesophagitis
- stomatitis
- herpes zoster.

Psychological and social support is provided by a team, who will provide support to the parents if the child is admitted to hospital or dies.

The carers should meet each month to discuss health and HIV education and how to give nutritional advice. Invited speakers, such as a professional nurse, a psychologist, nutritional experts or paediatricians could add value to the meetings. Social support programmes could include income-generating projects such as food stalls and handicrafts (*O'Hara et al. 2005*).

TRAINING HOME-BASED HEALTHCARE WORKERS

The training of home-based care workers could include the following:

- basic nursing care such as bed bathing, nail, hair and mouth care, pressure area care, general wound care and the handling of body fluids
- caring for the patient's environment such as bed making, changing linen, and general house cleaning

- assessing the nutritional needs of the patient and other family members in the household. Food may need to be prepared for the patient
- how to refer to other healthcare workers
- the treatment of HIV and AIDS-related conditions such as fever and diarrhoea, skin problems, nutritional problems, nausea, vomiting, pain and TB care
- information on community mobilisation and networking
- how to provide terminal care, the importance of confidentiality and respect for the patient and his/her condition
- how to deal with their own stress.

Community care workers need the following supplies:

- drugs per Disease Management and Control Guidelines, for pain control, and for control of other symptoms
- basic supplies (medical and assistive devices) – these may need to be improvised
- soap for hand washing and for washing the patient
- bandages, cotton wool, gauze and swabs, plasters and washable cloth
- disposable pads/incontinence sheets
- re-usable bedpans
- liquid bleach
- syringes and needles
- catheters, uro-bags and colostomy bags
- gloves and plastic aprons and bags for protection
- disinfectants for cleaning wounds
- small and medium plastic bags for soiled bandages and linen
- sugar, salt and rehydration solution and supplementary feeds, as well as infant feeds
- talcum powder for drying the skin after bathing.

(DOH 2001, Campbell 2004)

CONCLUSION

Home-based care calls upon the resources, skills, time and energy of communities, governments and funders. No single entity is able to meet the total requirements and challenges of home-based care for HIV and AIDS in South Africa today. A collaborative effort is needed and care in the community must become care by the community.

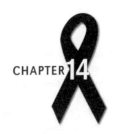

CHAPTER 14

PALLIATIVE CARE

Ansie Minnaar

> ## KEY CONCEPTS
>
> - symptom management
> - terminally ill
> - interdisciplinary team approach
> - living every day
> - hospice services
> - pain control, physical comfort, quality of life
> - alleviation of symptoms
> - analgesic ladder
> - pain symptoms
> - alternative pain relief
> - spiritual care
> - bereavement

Through my spirituality I give and receive love; I respond to and appreciate God, other people, a sunset, a symphony and spring.

(Stroll 1989, Kelly-Heidenthal 2003)

INTRODUCTION

Caring for dying people is often considered to be one of the more stressful aspects of nursing work, but can be very rewarding. Today, most terminally ill patients are cared for by hospice services. The term 'hospice' refers to a concept of humane and compassionate care, provided by an interdisciplinary team of professionals and delivered in a variety of settings:

- in a patient's home
- freestanding patient facilities
- nursing homes
- hospitals (*McKinnie & Kinzbrunner 2002*).

The hospice concept emphasises symptom management rather than disease-directed treatment, that is, quality rather than quantity of life. The terminally ill are comforted. An interdisciplinary team of professionals, including doctors, nurses, social workers, chaplains, home health aides, and others, provide comprehensive symptom management focusing on pain control and comfort measures as directed by the patient and family. Emotional, spiritual and practical support is given, based on the patient's and family's needs. Hospice is intended for patients with a life expectancy of six months or less. However, with good symptom management and pain control, many hospice patients live much longer. The key to hospice care is 'living every day' as patients prepare to die.

What hospice services can provide

Realistically, it is not possible for one person to meet all the needs of a seriously ill person and his/her family. Hospice services are provided by an interdisciplinary team. Members of the team work closely with each other, the patient and the family and meet weekly to coordinate care. Team members include the family doctor, nurse, home health aide, social worker, chaplain, volunteer, and the medical director.

The family doctor remains in charge of the patient's care, prescribes medications and closely consults with the hospice nurse. The nurse provides professional and skilled care and emotional support to the patient, family or significant others. The home health aide provides assistance with the basic needs of the patient such as bathing and personal care between one and seven times a week, during visits that last approximately one to two hours, depending on the needs of the patient/family/significant other. Tasks include: assistance with bed, tub or shower/bath, hair care, mouth care, and skin care as directed by the nurse, changing bed linen and keeping a neat patient area, assistance with meals as needed, assistance with elimination as directed by the nurse and emotional support to the patient/family/significant other.

When considering pain control look at physical, emotional and spiritual factors. Frequently, physical comfort cannot be achieved if the patient is experiencing severe emotional or spiritual distress or confusion. It is also true that a patient cannot address emotional or spiritual issues if he/she is in severe physical distress (*McKinnie & Kinzbrunner 2002*).

PRINCIPLES OF PALLIATIVE CARE

The overall goal of treatment is to optimise quality of life by helping to fulfill the hopes and desires of the patient. Death is regarded as a natural process, and is not hastened nor is life prolonged. Diagnostic tests and other invasive procedures are minimised, unless the results are likely to be useful in alleviating symptoms. When using narcotic analgesics, the 'right dose' is the dose that provides pain relief without unacceptable side effects. The patient is the expert on whether pain and other symptoms have been adequately relieved. Patients eat if they are hungry, and drink if they are thirsty; fluids and feeding are not forced. Care is individualised and based on the goals of the patient and family as the unit of care (McKinnie & Kinzbrunner 2002).

Pain management

The primary care doctor, with assistance from the hospice team, will determine the source of the pain and its treatment. Pain may be caused by factors related to the primary disease or by muscle spasm, constipation and poor position.

The World Health Organisaion principles of pain management include:

- *By the mouth:* Use oral agents whenever possible. Reserve alternative routes for patients who cannot take oral medication.
- *By the clock:* Patients with chronic pain require regular medication to prevent pain from occurring.
- *By the ladder:* See the WHO Analgesic Ladder below.
- *For the individual:* There is no specific dose of analgesic that is correct. Each patient must be medicated individually based on his/her individual needs (McKinnie & Kinzbrunner 2002).

The WHO Analgesic Ladder

The WHO Analgesic Ladder is an easy way to determine the correct analgesic. Each step in the ladder is defined by the severity of pain at presentation, which is rated on a scale of one to ten, with 0 representing the absence of pain and 10 being the most severe pain imaginable. There are three steps to the WHO Analgesic Ladder:

- step 1. Mild pain (severity 1-3) - Non-narcotic analgesics
- step 2. Moderate pain (severity 4-6) - Morphine-like agonists
- step 3. Severe pain (severity 7-10) - Morphine preparations.

Pain in HIV and AIDS patients

Peripheral neuropathy: This is one of the most common causes of pain or discomfort and narcotics alone may not be adequately effective.

Headache: Causes of headache include cryptococcosis, toxoplasmosis, lymphoma, and sinusitis.

Oral symptoms: These are usually caused by candidiasis (thrush). Use nystatin suspension five times daily.

Chest pain: This may be caused by esophogitis due to candida, herpes virus, or acid reflux. Treat the cause to relieve the pain.

Rectal pain: This may have a variety of causes. Investigate the possibility of herpes virus infection. Treat with topical analgesics or narcotics if required.

Neurologic symptoms: Find the cause of the symptoms. Headache may be caused by brain lesions or meningitis. Raised intracranial pressure may be relieved by serial lumbar puncture.

If depression is a significant factor in pain, use low-dose tricyclic antidepressants (*McKinnie & Kinzbrunner 2002*).

Alternative pain relief

We often think of medication as the single most important agent in the relief of pain. However, there are numerous other techniques and/or therapies that can decrease pain.

Distraction is often used as a way to stop thinking about pain. This can be as simple as listening to the radio or audio tapes/CDs, writing, reading, or even daydreaming.

Meditation is a conscious effort to relax our minds and body. For some, prayer achieves this state effectively. For others, such activities as yoga or tai chi, and imagery are effective ways of relaxing.

Hydrotherapy can be as simple as a relaxing bath or warm shower. Whirlpool baths or hot tubs are not always available, but a gentle form of hydrotherapy can be achieved by filling the bathtub, then allowing the water to run continuously as the tub drains. This process will keep water movement constant and provide a refreshing whirlpool effect.

Music is enjoyed by most people and can act as soothing therapy and a person's favorite music can provide a relaxing and therapeutic means of distraction. There are many commercially produced audio and/or video tapes, and CDs available specifically for relaxation therapy.

Humour is a very important stress releaser and motivator when coping with a difficult situation. It can help to break tension when nothing else will. Humour comes in many forms, funny videos or movies, and old stories.

Other symptom relief

Anorexia: Look for treatable reasons for loss of appetite first. If none are found, then try stimulating appetite by providing small, well-presented meals whenever the patient feels like eating. Add vitamin supplements if necessary. Sometimes a small alcoholic drink, such as a glass of sherry, will stimulate appetite.

Diarrhoea: Look for treatable causes of diarrhoea. Otherwise, use antidiarrhoeal agents such as lomotil as required.

Cough/dyspnoea: If this is caused by infection, then treat. If caused by intractable lung conditions, narcotic analgesics can relieve cough and breathlessness.

Spiritual care: Some patients may find that a spiritual approach to their illness is helpful. This may be faith based, or simply an appreciation of something outside oneself. Aspects of spirituality include accepting oneself, relating to others and relationships between and within groups (*Mahlangulu & Uys 2004*).

Bereavement and beyond: One of the most useful features of the hospice programme is bereavement follow up. Because patients and their families are special, the relationship with the family continues even after the patient's death.

Remember that nursing and other medical staff are also affected by a patient's death and may need help when a patient dies.

CONCLUSION

Providing good palliative care can be enormously rewarding. It requires careful attention to the patient's medical and emotional needs and is not simply about pain and symptom control. The best palliative care is provided by an integrated team that should include the patient's family and close friends.

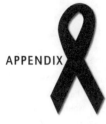

APPENDIX

OVERVIEW OF THE EPIDEMIOLOGY OF HIV

Candice Bodkin

KEY CONCEPTS

- epidemiology of HIV
- prevalence and incidence of HIV and AIDS
- projected consequences of HIV and AIDS
- South African approach to the management
- policies

INTRODUCTION

HIV and AIDS statistics supplied by the Medical Research Council in 2004 reveal a rather daunting scenario (*Ramjee 2005*). During 2004, approximately five million adults and children became HIV infected across the world. By the end of 2004, approximately 39.4 million people worldwide were living with HIV and AIDS. By 2004, an estimated three million people had died of AIDS.

HIV AND AIDS – THE REALITY

HIV and AIDS in sub-Saharan Africa

Sub-Saharan Africa is the region most affected by HIV and AIDS. It was estimated that by 2004, 25.4 million people were infected by HIV and AIDS. An estimated 3.1 million new infections occurred in sub-Saharan Africa in 2004. Two million children under the age of 15 years were expected to be living with HIV and AIDS in the region in 2004. A further 12 million children have been orphaned by HIV and AIDS. Approximately 90% of the children infected with HIV live in Africa. Of infants infected with HIV, approximately

15% die within two years of birth, an additional 75% die by age ten and only 10% live for ten years or longer.

HIV and AIDS in South Africa

In South Africa in 2004, it was estimated that 5.1 million people were living with HIV and AIDS. The majority (2.9 million) of HIV infections are found in women. Of children under 15 years, 230 000 are expected to be HIV positive. By 2005, it was estimated that 19% of adults in South Africa were infected with HIV (*Nattrass 2005*).

Despite the provision of antiretroviral therapy at selected public sector hospitals in South Africa (since April 2004), more and more HIV-infected people are now dying of AIDS. As a result the toll of AIDS will continue to rise, with devastating social and economic consequences.

In 2004 the Medical Research Council reported that HIV prevalence is the highest in KwaZulu-Natal (*Ramjee 2005*). The prevalence rate of HIV infection in KwaZulu-Natal ranges from 35% to 46% among non-pregnant women; the highest rates found in peri-urban areas and the lowest in rural areas. The HIV prevalence among pregnant women in KwaZulu-Natal is reported to be approximately 40.7%.

In 2004 the Reproductive Health Research Unit in Johannesburg revealed that 15.5% of adolescent girls (aged 15–21 years) were HIV positive. A similar study in the Western Cape showed an HIV prevalence of 5.9% among 15 to19-year-olds. A survey among 24 children's homes in Johannesburg in 2004 revealed an HIV prevalence of 25% (*Ramjee 2005*).

The progression of the HIV and AIDS epidemic in South Africa

The progression of the HIV and AIDS epidemic in South Africa can be described as four waves:

Wave 1

Wave 1 describes the incidence of HIV in South Africa, which peaked in 1998, with 930 000 new infections per year.

Wave 2

Wave 2 describes HIV prevalence in South Africa. Prevalence refers to the total number of people infected with HIV at any one time, and the peak is predicted to occur in 2006, at seven to eight million HIV infections. This prediction is made assuming no intervention for the treatment of HIV and AIDS.

Wave 3

The third wave describes deaths due to AIDS. AIDS-related deaths in South Africa are expected to peak in 2010, at 800 000 per year.

Wave 4

Wave 4 describes the peak in number of AIDS orphans in South Africa. The number of AIDS orphans is expected to peak in 2015, at approximately 1.85 million.

HIV and AIDS in South Africa: a socio-economic crisis

An overall adult prevalence of 19% amounts to a socio-economic crisis. This high HIV and AIDS infection rate reduces productivity, as economically active adults are becoming sick and dying, leaving behind orphans and the aged. A further complicating factor is that the HIV and AIDS epidemic in South Africa is occurring at a time when many South Africans are unemployed.

HIV AND AIDS AND MORTALITY

Mortality statistics from South African hospitals suggest that HIV-positive patients accounted for 44.9% of hospital deaths in 2004. Deaths among HIV-positive patients are primarily due to pulmonary and extrapulmonary tuberculosis, cryptococcal meningitis, pneumonia, *Pneumocystis jiroveci* and gastroenteritis (*Ramjee 2005*).

HIV AND PREGNANCY IN SOUTH AFRICA

The maternal mortality rate in South Africa is 150 per 100 000 maternities. The maternal mortality rate in the United Kingdom is 12.2 per 100 000 maternities. The high maternal mortality rate in South Africa can be attributed to the high incidence of non-pregnancy related infections that have become the leading cause of maternal mortality in South Africa since 1999. Non-pregnancy-related infections include: HIV and AIDS, pneumonia, tuberculosis, appendicitis, urinary tract infection, meningitis and malaria. The HIV and AIDS-related maternal mortality is likely to be underestimated as the HIV status was unknown in 64.5% of deaths.

Antenatal HIV statistics in South Africa indicate that HIV seroprevalence among pregnant women increased from 7.6% to 26.5% over the seven years, 1996–2003. HIV and AIDS in pregnancy places an added burden on the physical ability of the woman's body to cope with pregnancy. As a result,

HIV and AIDS during pregnancy causes an exaggeration of the problems related to pregnancy.

MANAGEMENT OF THE HIV AND AIDS CRISIS IN SOUTH AFRICA

HIV and AIDS has been identified as a national health priority since 1994 and is addressed within the National Health Plan for South Africa. The HIV/AIDS/STI Strategic Plan for South Africa (2000–2005) was launched in January 2000. This plan advocates the comprehensive management of HIV and AIDS, the provision of antiretroviral therapy and the prevention of mother-to-child transmission (PMTCT) of HIV. The management of HIV and AIDS in pregnancy and in adults generally involves triple therapy with antiretroviral therapy or highly active antiretroviral therapy (HAART). The antiretroviral therapy (first-line regimen) recommended for use in public sector hospitals in South Africa includes: stavudine, lamivudine, and efavirenz (*Wilson et al. 2002*).

Nevirapine (200 mg) administered at the onset of labour for the PMTCT of HIV has been provided to patients in certain public sector hospitals since March 2002.

In August 2003, Cabinet announced a plan for the 'roll-out' of free antiretrovirals for HIV-infected South Africans in public sector hospitals. As of July 2005 about 70 000 HIV-positive individuals were receiving antiretroviral therapy at public sector hospitals.

Provision of antiretrovirals in the public sector is a challenge. Doctors and nurses need to be trained in their use and patients need careful monitoring and follow up. This training is now being provided, both at medical and nursing schools and by private organisations. However, in addition to problems with the administration of antiretrovirals, public sector hospitals are finding it difficult to cope with the added burden of HIV infection. These challenges remain at the time of writing.

BIBLIOGRAPHY

Abrahams, N., Jewkes, R. & Mvo, Z. 2001. Health care-seeking practices of pregnant women and the role of the midwife in Cape Town, South Africa. *Journal of Midwifery and Women's Health*. 46: 240-247.

Afessa, B. & Green, B. 2000. Clinical course, prognostic factors, and outcome prediction for HIV patients in ICU: The PIP (Pulmonary Complications, ICU Support and Prognostic Factors in Hospitalised Patients with HIV) study. *Chest*. 118: 138-145.

Avidan, M.S., Jones, N. & Pozniak, A.L. 2000. The implications of HIV for the anaesthetist and the intensivist. *Anaesthesia*. 55: 344-354.

Baleta, A. 2003. South Africa stalls again on access to HIV drugs. *Lancet*. 361: 842.

Bartlett, J. G. & Gallant, J. E. 2000. *Medical Management of HIV Infection*. Baltimore: Johns Hopkins University.

Barrett-Grant, K., Fine, D., Heywood, M. & Strode, A. 2001. *HIV and AIDS and the Law*. Cape Town: The AIDS Law Project and the AIDS Legal Network.

Barrett-Grant, K., Strode, A & Smart, R. 2002. *Managing HIV and AIDS in the workplace:Aa guide for Government Departments*. Pretoria: The Department of Health Service and Administration.

Bhagwanjee, S., Muckart, D.J.J., Jeena, P.M. & Moodley, P. 1997. Does HIV status influence the outcome of patients admitted to a surgical intensive care unit? A prospective double blind study. *British Medical Journal*. 314: 1077-1081.

Bodkin, C. & Bruce, C. 2003. Health professional's knowledge of prevention strategies and protocol following percutaneous injuries. *Curationis*. 26(4): 22-28.

Bodkin, C., Klopper, H. & Langley, G. 2006. A comparison of HIV positive and negative pregnant women at a public sector hospital in South Africa. *Journal of Clinical Nursing* (15).

Brabin, B.J., Alexander, F.K. & Brown, N. 2003. Do disturbances within the folate pathway contribute to low birth weight in malaria? *Trends in Parasitology*.19: 39-44.

Butchart, A. & Villaveces, A. 2003. Violence against women and the risk of infant and child mortality. *Bulletin of the World Health Organisation*. I81: 17-19.

Cambell, S. 2004. Care of HIV/AIDS patients in developing countries. *Primary Health Care*. 13: 22-26.

Churchyard, G.J. & Metcalf, C. 2005. 2nd South African AIDS Conference report: Track 1: Basic and clinical sciences. *The South African Journal of HIV Medicine*. September 2005: 10-12

Cotton, M.F. 2005. Classification of HIV disease in children. *The South African Journal of HIV Medicine*. November 2005: 14-17

Craven, D.E. 1996. Symposium: Nosocomial colonization. Nosocomial colonization and infection in persons infected with human immunodeficiency virus. *Infection Control and Hospital Epidemiology*. 17: 304-318.

Cronje, H.S. & Grobler, C.J.F. 2003: *Obstetrics in Southern Africa*. Pretoria: Van Schaik.

Davies, S., Schneider, M., Rapholo, G. & Everatt, D. 1997. *Guidelines for developing a workplace policy and programme on HIV and AIDS and STIs*. Pretoria: DOH.

Department of Health. 2000. *HIV/AIDS/STI Strategic Plan for South Africa, 2000-2005*. Pretoria: DOH.

Department of Health. 2000. *Guidelines for Maternity Care in South Africa*. Pretoria: DOH.

Department of Health. 2002. *National HIV and syphilis sero-prevalence survey of women attending public antenatal clinics in South Africa*. http://www.doh.gov.za/docs/reports/2000/hivreport.html (Accessed April 2006).

Department of Health. 2001. *National Guideline on home-based care/community-based care*. Compiled by the Directorate, Chronic Diseases, Disabilities and Geriatrics. Pretoria: DOH.

Department of Health. 2002. *Summary Report: National HIV and Syphilis Antenatal Sero-prevalence Survey in South Africa, 2002*. Pretoria: DOH.

Department of Health. 2004. *National Antiretroviral Treatment Guidelines*. Pretoria: DOH.

Department of Health of South Africa, Gauteng Provincial Government. *Guidelines for the prophalaxis for accidential exposure to blood borne pathogens*. Pages 1-10. Pretoria: Government Printers.

De Visser, R., Ezzy, D. & Bartos, M. 2000. Alternative or complementary? Non-allopathic therapies for HIV/AIDS. *Alternative Therapies Health Medicine*. 6: 599-606.

De Visser, R. & Grierson, J. 2002. Use of alternative therapies by people living with HIV/AIDS in Australia. *AIDS Care*. 14:599-606.

Divine, B.T., Greby, S.M., Hunt, K.V., Kamb, M.L., Steketee, R.W. & Warner, L. 2001. *Revised Guidelines for HIV Counseling, testing and referral*. Technical Expert panel Review of CDC Counseling, Testing and Referral Guidelines. November 9, 2001 / 50 (RR19): 1-58. http://www.cdc.gov/mmwr/preview/mmwrhtml/rr5019a1.htm (Accessed April 2006).

Duse, A.G. 1999. Nosocomial infections in HIV-infected /AIDS patients. *Journal of Hospital Infection*. 43: 191-201.

Dye, T.R. 1995: *Understanding Public Policy*. Englewood, N.J: Prentice Hall.

Ehlers, V. 2002. Republic of South Africa: Policies and Politics Guide Nurses' Application of Genetic Technology in Public Health Settings. *Policy, Politics and Nursing Practice*. 3: 149-159.

Elion, R.A. & Cohen, C. 1997. Complementary medicine & HIV infection. *Primary Care*. 24(4): 905-919.

Ellis, J., Williams, H.W., Graves, W. & Lindsay, M.K. 2002. Human immunodeficiency virus infection is a risk factor for adverse perinatal outcome. *American Journal of Obstetrics and Gynaecology*. 186: 903-906.

Fan, H., Conner, R.F. & Villarreal, L.P. 2000. *AIDS science and society*. Third edition. Boston: Jones and Bartlett Publishers.

Fonchinggong, C.C., Mbuagbo, T.O., Abong, J.T. 2004. Barriers to counselling support for HIV/AIDS patients in South-Western Cameroon. *African Journal of AIDS Research*. 3: 157-163.

Farnham, P.G., Pinkerton, S.D., Holtgrave, D.R., Johnson-Masotti, A.P. 2002: *Cost-effectiveness of counselling and testing to prevent sexual transmission of HIV in the United States*. Vol 6(1): 33-43.

Freeman, J. 2003. *Toolkit: Managing HIV and AIDS in the workplace*. Pretoria: Services Seta.

Gardner, A. & Sibthorpe, B. 2002. Will he get back to normal? Survival and functional status after intensive care therapy. *Intensive and Critical Care Nursing*. 18: 139-145.

Grant, A.D. & De Cock, K.M. 2001. HIV and AIDS infection in the developing world. ABC of AIDS. *British Medical Journal*. 322: 1475-1478.

Griffis, D.I., Delate, T. & Coons, S. J. 2001. Predictors of mental (MHS) and physical (PHS) health summary scores of the MOS-HIV in a sample of HIV infected patients. *Value in Health*. 4: 131.

Harrison, A., Smit, J.A., Myer, L. 2000. Prevention of HIV/AIDS in South Africa: A review of behaviour change interventions, evidence and options for the future. *South African Journal of Science*. 96: 285-290.

Hathcock, A.L., Silverman, P., Ferre, C., Reynolds, M.A., Schieve, L.A. & Drees, M. 2003: Increasing infant mortality among very low birth weight infants – Delaware, 1994-2000. *Morbidity and Mortality Weekly Report*. 52: 862-866.

Henderson, C.W. 2001. HIV patients use CAM very often without physician knowledge. *AIDS Weekly*. 06/04/2001.

HIV/AIDS Update 2004: Orlando Regional Healthcare, Education & Development.

Hsiao, A.F., Wong, M.D., Kanouse, D.E., Collins, R.L., Honghu, L., Andersen, R.M., Grifford, A.L., McCutchan, A.B., Samuel, A., Shapiro, M.F. & Wenger, N.S. 2003. Complementary and Alternative Medicine Use and Substitution for Conventional Therapy by HIV-Infected Patients. *Journal of Acquired Immune Deficiency Syndromes*. 33: 157-166.

International Association of Physicians in AIDS care (IAPAC). 2005. *Clinical Guidelines for Antiretroviral Therapy in Adults*. http://www.iapac.org. (Accessed April 2006).

Jones, R. & Nelson, M. 2005. New strategies and novel antiretroviral therapies for the treatment of HIV infection. *The South African Journal of HIV Medicine*. September 2005: 18–25.

Kelly-Heidenthal, P. 2003. *Nursing Leadership and management*. New York: Thomson Delmar Learning.

Khouli, H., Afrasiabi, A., Shibli, M., Hajal, R., Redington-Barrett, C. & Homel, P. 2005. Outcome of critically ill human immunodeficiency virus-infected patients in the era of highly active antiretroviral therapy. *Journal of Intensive Care Medicine*. 20: 327–285.

Kinghorn, S. & Gamlin, R. 2001. *Palliative Nursing: Bring comfort and hope*. London: Bailliere Tindall.

Kjell, H., Mortensen, J.H.S. & Wollen, A. 2003. Preterm delivery: an overview. *Acta Obstetrica et Gynecologica Scandinavica*. 82: 687–705.

Knipples, H.M. & Weiss, J.J. 2000. Use of alternative medicine in a sample of HIV positive gay men: an exploratory study of prevalence and user characteristics. *AIDS Care*. 12: 435–446.

Kumar, P. & Clark, D. 2004. *Clinical Medicine*. Fifth edition. London: Saunders.

Laing, R.B.S. 1999. Nosocomial infections in patients with HIV disease. *Journal of Hospital Infection*. 43:170–185.

Ledwaba, L. 2005. South Africa: Home-based care a critical need where 1 in 5 have HIV. *The New York Amsterdam News*. December 15–21: 2.

Lucas, S. 2001. Update on the pathology of AIDS. *Intensive and Critical Care Nursing*. 17: 155–166.

Madsen, H., Anderson, S., Nielsen, R.G., Dolmer, B.S., Host, A. & Damkier, A. 2003. The use of complementary and alternative medicine among paediatric patients. *European Journal of Paediatrics*. 162: 334–342.

Madhaven, S. 2004: Fosterage patterns in the age of AIDS: continuity and change. *Social Science Medicine*. 58:1443–1445.

Mahlangulu S.N. & Uys, L.R. 2004. Spirituality in nursing: An analysis of the concept. *Curationis*. 27: 15–26.

Marchal, B., De Brouwere, V. & Kegels, G. 2005. HIV and AIDS and the health workforce crisis: What are the next steps? *Tropical medicine and International Health*. 10: 300–304.

Marriner-Tomey, A. 2004. *Guide to Nursing Management and Leadership*. 5th edition. St Louis: Mosby.

Mascolini, M. 2001. Viro-diversity: or, keeping up with HIV's evolutionary caprice. *5th International Workshop on HIV Drug Resistance and Treatment Strategies*. June 4–8, 2001. Arizona: Scottsdale.

Martinson, N., Hausler, H., Churchyard, G.J. & Lawn, S.D. 2003. Dealing with the dual epidemics of HIV and TB. *The South African Journal of HIV Medicine*. September 2003: 33–35.

Mckinnie, J. & Kinzbrunner, B. 2002. *HIV/AIDS primary care guide, Florida AIDS Education and Training Centre*. Florida: University of Florida.

Minnaar, A. 2005. HIV and AIDS issues in the workplace of nurses. *Curationis*. 28: 31-38.

Morris, A., Masur, H. & Huang, L. 2006: Current issues in critical care of the human immunodeficiency virus-infected patient. *Critical care Medicine*. 34: 41-49.

Morris, K. 2001. Treating HIV in South Africa - a tale of two systems. *The Lancet*. 357: 1190.

Morton, P.G., Fontaine, D., Hudak, C.M. & Gallo, B.M. 2005. *Critical Care Nursing: A Holistic Approach*. Eighth edition. Philadelphia: Lippincott.

Mubangizi, J. 2004. HIVand AIDS and the South African Bill of rights, with specific reference to the approach and role of the courts. *African Journal of AIDS research*. 3 : 113-119.

Nattress, N. 2005. AIDS, unemployment and disability in South Africa: The case for welfare reform. *The South African Journal of HIV Medicine*. September 2005.

O'Hare, B.A.M. Venables, J. Nalubeg, J.F. Nakakeeto, M. Kibirige, M. & Southall, D.P. 2005. Home-based care for orphaned children infected with HIV/AIDS in Uganda. *AIDS Care*. 17: 443-450.

Padoveze, M.C., Trabasso, P. & Branchini, M.L.M. 2002. Nosocomial infections among HIV-positive and HIV-negative patients in a Brazilian infectious diseases unit. *American Journal of Infection Control*. 30:346-350.

Patchen, L. & Beal, M.W. 2001. Preventing perinatal transmission of HIV: An evidence based update for midwives. *Journal of Midwifery and Women's Health*. 46: 354-363.

Patel, P., Best, B. & Capparelli, E.V. 2005. Paediatric antiretroviral pharmacology. *The South African Journal of HIV Medicine*. November 2005. 8-13.

Pattinson, R. C. 2000. *Saving babies: A perinatal care survey of South Africa: 2000 executive summary*. http://www.scienceinafrica.co.za/2001/july/babies.htm. 01/08/2003. (Accessed April 2006).

Peterson, K.P., Hunter, D. J. & Fawzi, W.W. 2002. Effect of multivitamin and vitamin A supplements on weight gain during pregnancy among HIV-infected women. *American Journal of Clinical Nutrition*. 75: 1082-1090.

Piscitelli, S.C. 2000. The use of complementary therapies by patients with HIV: Full sail into unchartered waters. *Medscape HIV/AIDS*. 6:1-6

Ramjee, G. 2005. Second South African AIDS conference report: Track 2. HIV Epidemiology, Prevention and Public Health. *The South African Journal of HIV Medicine*. September 2005.

Ramphele, M. 2005. HIV/AIDS: The Mirror in South Africa's face. *The South African Journal of HIV Medicine*. September 2005: 5-8.

Reid, G. 2002. Probiotics for urogenital health. *Nutrition in Clinical Care*. 5: 3-9.

Reznik, D.A. 2005. Oral manifestations of HIV disease. *Topics in HIV Medicine* 13: 143-148.

Rosen, S., Simon, J.L., Thea, D.M. & Vincent, J.R. 2000. Care and treatment to extend the working lives of HIV-positive employees: Calculating the benefits to business. *South African Journal of Science*. 96: 300-304.

Sengwana, M. 2005. Health care workers bear the burden of HIV and AIDS. *Nursing Update*. 29: 30.

Sidley, P. 2003a. South African Government to withdraw antiretrovirals for pregnant mothers. *British Medical Journal*. 327: 306-307.

Sidley, P. 2003b. Cabinet rules that South Africans must be given antiretrovirals. *British Medical Journal*. 327:357.

Slattery, M. M. & Morrison, J.J. 2002. Preterm delivery. *Lancet*. 360: 1489-1497.

Smit, R. 2005. HIV and AIDS and the workplace: Perceptions of nurses in a public hospital in South Africa. *Journal of Advanced Nursing*. 51: 22-29.

South Africa. 1993. *The Compensation for Occupational Injuries Act*. (Act 130 of 1993) Pretoria: Government Printer.

South Africa. 1995. *The Labour Relations Act*. (Act 66 of 1995). Pretoria: Government Printer.

South Africa. 1996. *The Occupational Health and Safety Act*. (Act 29 of 1996). Pretoria: Government Printer.

South Africa. 1996. *The South African Constitution Act*. (Act 108 of 1996). Pretoria: Government Printer.

South Africa. 1998. *The Employment Equity Act*. (Act 55 of 1998). Pretoria: Government Printer.

South Africa. 1998. *The Medical Schemes Act*. (Act 131 of 1998). Pretoria: Government Printer.

South Africa. 2000. *The Promotion of Equality and the Prevention of Unfair Discrimination Act*. (Act 4 of 2000) Pretoria: Government Printer.

South Africa. *The Code of Good Practice and Key Aspects of HIV and AIDS and Employment*. Unpublished.

South African Nursing Council. Regulation R2488. 26 October 1990.

Sowell, R.L. 2005. It's leadership - stupid! *Journal of the Association of Nurses in AIDS Care*. 16(1): 1-2.

Standish, L.J., Greene, K B., Bain, S., Reeves, C., Sanders, F., Wines, R C.M., Turret, P., Kim, J.G. & Calabrese, C. 2001. Alternative medicine usage in HIV positive men and women: Demographics, utilisation patterns and health status. *AIDS Care*. 13:197-208.

Stratton, P., Tuomala, R.E., Abboud, R., Rodriguez, E., Rich, K., Pitt, J., Diaz, C. & Hammill, H. 1999. Obstetric and newborn outcomes in a cohort of HIV-infected pregnant women: a report of the women and infant transmission study. *Journal of Acquired Immune Deficiency Syndromes and Human Retrovirology*. Vol. 20: 179-186.

Stroud, L., Srivastava, P., Culver, D., Bison, D., Rimland, D., Simberkoff, M., Elder, H., Fierer, J., Martone, W. & Gayness, R. 1997. Nosocomial infections in HIV-infected patients: Preliminary results from a multicentre surveillance system. *Infection Control and Hospital Epidemiology*. 18: 479-485.

Swanepoel, B., Erasmus, B. & Schenk, H. 2001. *South African Human Resource Management*. Cape Town: Juta.

The International Association of Physicians in AIDS Care and the South Africa HIV/AIDS Clinicians Society. www.iapac.org.

UNAIDS 2002. Report on the global HIV/AIDS epidemic. Geneva: UNAIDS.

UNAIDS 2004. Report on the global HIV/AIDS epidemic. Geneva: UNAIDS.

Uys, L.R. 2003. Aspects of the care of people with HIV/AIDS in South Africa. *Public Health Nursing*. 20: 271-280.

Venter, F.W.D. 2005. A critical evaluation of the *South African state antiretroviral programme*. The South African Journal of HIV Medicine. September 2005.

Villamor E., Saathoff E., Msamanga G., O'Brien M.E., Manji K., Fawzi W.W. 2005. Wasting during pregnancy increases the risk of mother-to-child HIV-1 transmission. *Journal of Acquired Immune Deficiency Syndrome* (38):622-6.

Walt, G. & Gilson, L. 1994. Reforming the Health Sector in Developing Countries: The Central Role of Policy Analysis. *Health Policy Planning Weekly*. 9: 353-370.

White, L. 2001. *Foundations of nursing care for the whole person*. Texas: Delmar.

Whiteside, A. 2000. The real challenges: The orphan generation and employment creation. *AIDS Analysis Africa*. 10:14-15.

Wilson, D., Naidoo, S., Bekker, L., Cotton, M. & Maartens, G. 2002. *Handbook of HIV Medicine*. Cape Town: Oxford University Press.

Ziady, L.E., Small, N. & Louis, A.M.J. 1997. *Rapid reference Infection Control*. Pretoria: Kagiso Tertiary.

A GLOSSARY OF HIV AND AIDS TERMS

AIDS	Acquired Immunodeficiency Syndrome – a syndrome (collection of diseases) that results from infection with the HI virus
Antibodies	Substances produced by cells in the body's immune system in response to foreign substances that have entered the body
Asymptomatic	Exhibiting no medical symptoms
Care	A broad term referring to the steps taken to promote a person's wellbeing through medical, psychosocial, spiritual and other means
Clinical trial	Research to determine the safety and efficacy of a new drug or treatment in humans
Confidentiality	The right of every person, employee or job applicant to have his or her medical information, including HIV status, kept private
ELISA test	Enzyme Linked ImmunoSorbent Assay – the test used to identify the presence or absence of HIV antibodies
Epidemic	A disease, usually infectious, that spreads quickly through a population
Epidemiology	The study of the distribution and determinants of disease in human populations
Evaluation	The assessment of the impact of a programme at a particular point in time
Health promotion	Programmes aimed at ensuring the physical and mental health and wellbeing of employees
HIV	Human immunodeficiency virus – the name of the virus, which undermines the immune system and leads to AIDS
HIV testing	Any form of testing designed to identify the HIV status of a person, including blood tests, saliva tests or medical questionnaires
Immune system	A complex system of cells and cell substances that protect the body from infection and disease
Incidence of HIV	The number of new cases of HIV in a given time period, often expressed as a percentage of the susceptible population

Monitoring	The systematic and continuous assessment of a programme over a period of time
Occupational exposure	Exposure to blood or other body fluids, which may be HIV infected, during the course of carrying out working duties (for example, a health-care worker may be exposed to HIV in the case of a needle stick injury)
Opportunistic infections	Infections that occur because a person's immune system is so weak that microorganisms that often do not normally cause disease, can cause disease
Pandemic	An epidemic occurring simultaneously in many countries
Policy	A document setting out a department's or organisation's position on a particular issue (for example, a policy setting out the steps to be taken following occupational exposure to HIV)
Positive living skills	Skills that empower people living with AIDS (PLWAs) to cope with the difficulties and challenges they might face, and to live a long and fulfilling life
Prevalence of HIV	The number of people with HIV at a point in time, often expressed as a percentage of the total population
Prevention programme	A programme designed to prevent HIV transmission, including components such as awareness, education and training, condom distribution, treatment of sexually transmitted infections, occupational infection control
Rapid HIV testing	An HIV testing process, which enables a test result to be achieved within 10 to 30 minutes
Seroconversion	The point at which the immune system produces antibodies and at which time the HIV antibody test can show an HIV infection
Support services	Assistance that could be provided to help a person deal with difficult situations and challenges
Treatment	A medical term describing the steps being taken to care for and manage an illness
Window period	The period between infection with HIV and seroconversion (when HIV antibodies can be detected by the HIV antibody test)

ACRONYMS AND ABBREVIATIONS

AIDS	Acquired Immunodeficiency Syndrome
CIDA	Canadian International Development Agency
CCMA	Commission for Conciliation, Mediation and Arbitration
DOH	Department of Health
DOTS	Directly Observed Treatment Short-course
EAP	Employee Assistance Programme
EIA	Enzyme immunoassays
FOSAD	Forum of South African Directors-General
GEPF	Government Employees' Pension Fund
HOD	Head of Department
HIV	Human Immunodeficiency Virus
HR	Human resources
HSRC	Human Sciences Research Council
IDC	Interdepartmental Committee on HIV/AIDS
ILO	International Labour Organisation
KAP	Knowledge, attitudes and practices
M&E	Monitoring and evaluation
MRC	Medical Research Council
MTEF	Medium-term Expenditure Framework
NAPWA	National Association of People living with HIV/AIDS
PEP	Post-exposure prophylaxis
PFMA	Public Finance Management Act
PHRC	Provincial Health Restructuring Committee
PLWA	Person living with HIV/AIDS
PMTCT	Prevention of mother-to-child transmission
PSCBC	Public Service Co-ordinating Bargaining Council
SACMA	South African Civil Military Alliance
SADC	Southern African Development Community
SAPS	South African Police Service

SANAC	South African National AIDS Council
SANDF	South African National Defence Force
SMS	Senior Management Service
STI	Sexually transmitted infection
TB	Tuberculosis
UNAIDS	Joint United Nations Programme on HIV/AIDS
USAID	United States Agency for International Development
VCT	Voluntary counselling and testing
WHO	World Health Organisation

INDEX